Mental Health
Problems and
Older Adults

Choices and Challenges:
An Older Adult Reference Series
Elizabeth Vierck, Series Editor

Housing Options and Services for Older Adults,
Ann E. Gillespie and Katrinka Smith Sloan

Mental Health Problems and Older Adults,
Gregory A. Hinrichsen

Paying for Health Care after Age 65,
Elizabeth Vierck

Forthcoming

Legal Issues and Older Adults,
Linda Josephson Millman and Sallie Birket Chafer

Older Workers, Sara E. Rix

Travel and Older Adults, Allison St. Claire

Volunteerism and Older Adults, Mary K. Kouri

Mental Health Problems and Older Adults

Gregory A. Hinrichsen, Ph.D.

Geropsychiatry Service and Research Department
Hillside Hospital, A Division of Long Island Jewish Medical Center
Assistant Professor of Psychiatry
Albert Einstein College of Medicine

Choices and Challenges: An Older Adult Reference Series
Elizabeth Vierck, Series Editor

ABC-CLIO

Santa Barbara, California
Oxford, England

Cover Design/Graphein

Library of Congress Cataloging-in-Publication Data

Hinrichsen, Gregory A., 1951–
    Mental health problems and older adults / Gregory A. Hinrichsen.
      p. cm.—(Choices and challenges)
    Includes bibliographical references and index.
    1. Aged—Mental health—Handbooks, manuals, etc. 2. Aged—Mental
health services—Handbooks, manuals, etc. I. Title. II. Series.
    RC451.4.A5H56   1990   618.97'689—dc20   90-40319

ISBN 0-87436-240-7 (alk. paper)

97 96 95 94 93 92 91 90   10 9 8 7 6 5 4 3 2 1

This book is not intended to provide medical advice nor intended to take the place of advice from a mental health professional. A competent professional should be consulted when mental health services appear to be needed.

ABC-CLIO, Inc.
130 Cremona Drive, P.O. Box 1911
Santa Barbara, California 93116-1911

Clio Press Ltd.
55 St. Thomas' Street
Oxford, OX1 1JG, England

This book is Smyth-sewn and printed on acid-free paper ∞ .
Manufactured in the United States of America

For Kay

Contents

Foreword, xi
Preface, xv
Acknowledgments, xix
How To Use This Book, xxi

PART ONE: **Mental Health Problems**

Chapter 1:   Mood Disorders, 3

Basic Facts, 3

Introduction, 5

Depression, 7
Definition, 7
Frequency, 13
Possible Causes, 14
Evaluation, 24
Treatment, 33
Effectiveness of Treatments, 56

Bipolar Disorder and Cyclothymia, 57
Definition, 57
Frequency and Possible Causes, 60
Evaluation, 61
Treatment, 61
Effectiveness of Treatments, 64

Mood Disorders and the Family, 65

Chapter 2:   Cognitive Problems, 67

Basic Facts, 67

Introduction, 68

Normal Aging of the Human Brain, 70

Abnormal Changes in the Brain, 71
Definitions of Cognitive Problems, 72
Frequency of Dementias and Delirium among Older Adults, 77
Causes of Delirium and Dementias, 78
Evaluation of Cognitive Problems, 85
Treatment of Cognitive Problems, 92
The Outcome of Cognitive Problems, 101

Chapter 3: **Other Mental Health Problems, 105**

Basic Facts, 105

Introduction, 109

Schizophrenia and Delusional Disorder, 110
Definition, 111
Frequency, 117
Possible Causes, 117
Evaluation, 119
Treatment, 119
Effectiveness of Treatments, 124

Anxiety Disorders, 125
Definition, 125
Frequency, 129
Possible Causes, 130
Evaluation, 130
Treatment, 131
Effectiveness of Treatments, 134

Substance Use Disorders, 135
Definition, 135
Frequency, 137
Possible Causes, 138
Evaluation, 140
Treatment, 142
Outcome of Substance Use Disorders in Late Life, 143

Chapter 4: **The Mental Health System and the Older Adult, 145**

Basic Facts, 145

Introduction, 146

Historical Perspectives on Care of Older Adults
with Mental Disorders, 147

The Present System of Mental Health Care for
Older Adults, 150
　　Outpatient Mental Health Care, 151
　　Inpatient Mental Health Services, 153

The Funding of Mental Health Care for Older
Adults, 154
　　Medicare, 154
　　Medicaid, 156
　　Private Insurance, 157

Problems in the Mental Health Care System for
Older Adults, 157
　　Financial Problems, 157
　　Training and Manpower Problems, 158
　　Coordination Problems among Service Systems, 159
　　Older People's Reluctance To Use Services, 160
　　Problems in Nursing Homes, 161

Practical Suggestions for Finding and Using
Mental Health Services, 162
　　How To Find Services, 162
　　How To Use Mental Health Services, 165

References for Part One, 171

PART TWO:　**Resources**

Chapter 5:　**Directory of Organizations, 175**

　　National Resources, 175

　　State and Local Resources, 188

Chapter 6:　**Reference Materials, 221**

　　Books, 221
　　　　Books for the Professional, 221
　　　　Books for the General Public, 228

　　Pamphlets, 235

　　Films and Videocassettes, 244

Glossary, 251

Appendix A: Alphabetic Listing of Psychotropic Medications
    by Generic and Trade Names, 263

Appendix B: Summary of Criteria for *DSM-III-R* Disorders,
    267

Index, 289

Foreword

Your prospective client has passed his eightieth birthday. Although he shows numerous signs of depression, you hesitate to make this diagnosis because there are several situational factors that are likely to be influencing his mood:

1. He is a refugee (actually, an escapee) from his homeland who fled under circumstances that intensify the stress one usually encounters in making such a major life change.
2. He is in constant pain from a life-threatening illness.
3. His energy has been depleted by undergoing a series of surgical procedures that have brought neither remission nor relief.
4. He is aware that he does not have long to live.
5. He is worried—and for good reason—about the safety and well-being of many of the important people in his life.

As you study his dossier, other problems become evident. The old man seems to have an "addictive personality." Although he apparently liberated himself from a drug addiction many years ago, he has never been able to conquer the craving for nicotine. Even now, in his frailty and anguish, he continues to smoke, knowing that this habit has contributed much to his physical decline. Along with all of the above, you draw the inference that he is a "difficult" person, hypersensitive and well defended. In all likelihood, he would be suspicious of your motives and dubious about your qualifications.

Given this prospect, what course of action would you take? Perhaps you would judge that he is a poor candidate for counseling or psychotherapy—as well as a "tough nut" who would reward your efforts with nothing but frustration. Perhaps you would recommend pharmacological intervention to modify his mood somewhat (but don't bother, he is stubbornly set even against taking pain medication). Perhaps you would think of hospitalizing him for his own good—and, along with that, why not a course of electroconvulsive shock treatments if his physical health can bear it? Any of these options could seem more practical and appealing than committing yourself to establishing a therapeutic relationship with this cranky old wreck.

But, then again, you might decide that Sigmund Freud was still a fascinating and valuable fellow. You might find yourself admiring the stubborn streak that impels him to reject any medication that might dull his mind and interfere with his continuing work. You might find yourself respecting his all-too-human quirks and the emotional scars that have formed over his lifelong inner conflicts. Are these not the appropriate emblems and medals for a person who mined his own anxieties to produce a powerful if controversial new perspective on human nature? Would you really want to miss this opportunity to know and perhaps help Dr. Freud because he is supposedly too old to benefit from psychological intervention? (And perhaps also you would miss his mature reflections on his own earlier contention that elderly people would not benefit from therapy!)

Admittedly, we are not likely to encounter a Sigmund Freud among prospective clients as we go about our responsibilities as psychologist, psychiatrist, social worker, pastoral counselor, or other human services provider. But we are likely to encounter many elderly men and women who are experiencing anxiety, depression, memory loss, and a variety of other disturbances. How prepared do we find ourselves for these encounters? Have we managed to free ourselves from pervasive cultural stereotypes that portray older adults as either used-up machines or "poor little dears" who cannot be expected to do much for themselves? And have we equipped our minds with the best available knowledge regarding mental health and illness in the later adult years?

Gregory Hinrichsen has now made it much easier for mental health professionals to bring themselves up to speed in assessing the mental health status of elderly adults and designing effective preventive and interventive actions. To this valuable task he brings his own considerable clinical experience as well as his command of the rapidly growing scholarly and professional literature in gerontology/geriatrics. He is a trustworthy guide who, through his book, fulfills his promise to lead readers through the basics. Having read this book, those with particular interests and responsibilities in the care of elderly adults will be in a better position to pursue the current literature on specific topics.

The very existence of this book attests to the substantial progress that has been made in recent years. Back in—could it really have been *that* long ago?—well, never mind the date! But when I was the latest model of the Ph.D. in clinical psychology, the expectation that I might research or conduct therapy with elderly adults was near zero. My knowledge on that topic also hovered on the near-zero level. Along with a small, scattered, but gradually accumulating number of other practitioners and sociobehavioral scientists, I did discover that older men and women were a source of almost unlimited surprise, challenge, and reward, even—or especially—when they were confronting some of life's darkest moments. There's no doubt that I would have made many mistakes and false starts even if a book such as this one had been available at that time. But there is also no doubt that I would have benefited from the knowledge and guidance Hinrichsen provides to us all. In turn, Hinrichsen's own contribution is possible because many others have also rejected nihilistic stereotypes and made their clear-eyed and valuable observations.

The author provides us with a wealth of up-to-date information about mental illness in later life. This material and the author's own observations should help to reduce the hesitancies and emotional barriers that have too often interfered with the mental health service provider's response to the troubled older person. What has been left out, then? I suggest that we all need to be more aware of the positive aspects of mental health in later life. Many men and women bring ripe experiences and well-honed skills to their later years, enjoy life immensely, and contribute much to the diversity and quality of our society. I feel pretty sure that the author would agree with the proposition that health is not simply the absence of illness. And now you have completed your unusually diligent action (I mean, who reads forewords, anyway?), and this timely and useful book itself awaits your attention.

Robert Kastenbaum, Ph.D.
Department of Communication
Arizona State University

Preface

In the planning stages of this book I told the series editor that I hoped I might be fortunate enough to get Robert Kastenbaum to write the foreword. He is not only a pioneer in the field of mental health and aging but also has been a source of inspiration to many of us because of his passionate commitment to the human dimensions of gerontology and geriatrics. I am grateful to Dr. Kastenbaum for writing a lively and provocative foreword.

As Dr. Kastenbaum notes in the foreword, however, a book on this topic runs some dangers. By focusing on problems of older adults we may inadvertently contribute to the image of all older people as frail, depleted, and trouble-ridden. He rightly reminds us that many older people lead satisfying lives to which they bring many assets developed through long years of experience. By delineating the usual treatments provided by professionals to older "patients," we may fail to communicate the considerable personal satisfaction that mental health workers may gain from assisting older people with problems and how older people themselves may teach their helpers important lessons on how to meet the often complex issues of getting older. Dr. Kastenbaum's playful case of an older adult who just happens to be the famous Sigmund Freud challenges all of us to better grapple with the larger meanings of even the most annoying and perplexing symptoms of older clients. For these symptoms may be important clues in understanding the richness and beauty of lives lived long.

There have been many advances in the mental health field in the last 20 years. Pharmacological treatments of major mental disorders have been refined and expanded. Psychological treatments have grown more sophisticated. Our understanding of the biological underpinnings of mental illness has grown rapidly. Despite these advances, research on and treatments for the mental health problems of older adults have developed more slowly. Easy access for older adults to affordable mental health services provided by well-trained professionals is more a goal than a reality.

Professionals interested in familiarizing themselves with mental health and aging fortunately will find several excellent texts on the diagnosis and treatment of major mental disorders in older adults. Many of these books are written by psychiatrists and assume that the reader is generally familiar with current issues in psychiatric diagnosis, common medical problems of late life, and psychopharmacological treatment of major mental disorders. Before reading one or several of these books, however, some mental health professionals may initially desire a general orientation to the major psychiatric, psychological, and psychosocial issues that bear on mental health problems and aging. This may be especially true for those without medical training or those who are less familiar with recent developments in the mental health field. It is the intention of this book to fill that need.

Older people and/or their families may also want to gain familiarity with major issues in the diagnosis and treatment of late life mental disorders. Frequently this is the case when an older adult and/or the family feel that an evaluation for mental health problems may be needed. At present, information for the general public on many topics of mental health problems and aging is not readily available.

The first section of this book discusses major issues in the nature, frequency, diagnosis, treatment, and prognosis of the most common mental health problems that affect older adults. Chapter 1 reviews these issues as they bear on late life mood disorders. Chapter 2 examines cognitive problems. Chapter 3 discusses a variety of other mental health problems that may affect older people, including schizophrenia and delusional disorder, anxiety disorders, and substance use disorders. Chapter 4 addresses past and current issues in the delivery of mental health services to older adults and offers some practical suggestions for consumers of mental health services on how to find and utilize those services.

The first three chapters contain clinical vignettes based on my professional work with older adults over the last 12 years. The vignettes derive from work as a geriatric social service outreach worker in Boston, as a researcher at Hillside Hospital on family issues in late life mental disorders, and as a staff psychologist at Hillside Hospital's outpatient geriatric mental health program. The names used in the vignettes are fictitious, and any identifying information has been changed. The vignettes, however, convey the substance of actual mental health problems confronted by older adults and their families.

The second part of *Mental Health Problems and Older Adults* is a resource section designed for readers seeking further information on mental health and aging or on mental health services. The information provided includes:

- A listing of national organizations concerned with aging, mental health, or mental health and aging. An effort was made to ascertain whether these organizations would be able to provide help to people trying to locate services for older adults.

- State and local resources, including lists of state or regional offices of mental health and aging organizations that may be contacted by those seeking information about area services or self-help groups.

- Reference materials, including an annotated bibliography of a select group of books and an annotated listing of pamphlets available from different organizations.

- A review of selected current films and videocassettes on mental health and aging.

- A glossary for those seeking brief definitions of concepts that are discussed in the book.

- An appendix with an alphabetical listing of psychotropic medications by both generic and trade names.

- An appendix with the complete *Diagnostic and Statistical Manual of Mental Disorders* (*DSM-III-R*) criteria for mental disorders that are reviewed in this book (reproduced with permission of the American Psychiatric Association).

In recent years people with mental health problems and their families have evidenced a growing interest in becoming more knowledgeable and active consumers of mental health care. This is evident in the rapid growth of a variety of mental health self-help and advocacy groups. A fundamental premise of these groups is that knowledge empowers people to find the best available mental health resources, motivates individuals to be active participants in their mental health care, and stimulates people to lobby for better mental health research and services. In the field of aging, the remarkable growth and influence of the Alzheimer's Association well demonstrates the active role that can be played by families of people seriously affected by mental disorders. Such efforts perhaps herald the beginning of a new and more mature relationship between people who receive mental health services and those who provide them. It is hoped that this book will contribute to the further development of that relationship.

Gregory A. Hinrichsen

Acknowledgments

Professional colleagues and friends have contributed to completion of this book. Blaine Greenwald, M.D., and Bruce Saltz, M.D., offered substantive comments on various chapters. Robert Jerome, a communications consultant and friend, provided valuable stylistic advice. Joan L. Kauff, Lenore Letterman, and Lillian T. Buller of the Hillside Hospital Health Sciences Library offered considerable assistance in identifying and retrieving primary research materials. Arlene Cohen, A.C.S.W., and Leonard Tuzman, A.C.S.W., provided useful suggestions regarding the book's resource section. Adrienne Grande assisted with the process of assembling research materials, and Lori Manzano, with typing parts of the manuscript.

Elizabeth Vierck, editor of the series of which this book is a part, provided the original impetus for this project and offered helpful advice throughout its course. In addition to being a professional colleague, she is a friend of almost 20 years. Laurie Brock ably guided the manuscript through the publication process at ABC-CLIO.

Special thanks to clinical colleagues and teachers from past and present from whom I have learned much about the process of helping older people. Marjorie Glassman, A.C.S.W., and Jane Eckert, A.C.S.W., taught me early lessons about mental health and aging in Boston's Fenway neighborhood. Barbara J. Felton, Ph.D., my academic mentor at New York University, showed me the methods and value of scholarship. Allen Willner, Ph.D., has offered practical and compassionate guidance in my clinical work at Hillside Hospital's outpatient mental health clinic for older adults. Kathy Byrne, Ph.D., a clinical gerontology colleague and friend, has generously shared her experience and insights on doing psychotherapy with older adults.

How To Use This Book

Each book in the Choices and Challenges series provides a convenient, easy-access reference tool on a specific topic of interest to older adults and those involved with them, including caregivers, spouses, adult children, and gerontology professionals. The books are designed for ease of use, with a generous typeface, ample use of headings and subheadings, and a detailed index.

Each book consists of two parts, which may be used together or independently:

A narrative section providing an informative and comprehensive overview of the topic, written for a lay audience. The narrative can be read straight through or consulted on an as-needed basis by using the headings and subheadings and/or the index.

An annotated resource section that includes a directory of relevant organizations; recommended books, pamphlets, and articles; and software and videos. Where appropriate, the resource section may include additional information relevant to the topic. This section can be used in conjunction with or separately from the narrative to locate sources of additional information, assistance, or support.

A glossary defines important terms and concepts, and the index provides additional access to the material. For easy reference, entries in the resource section are indexed by both topic and title or name.

PART ONE

Mental Health
Problems

Chapter 1

Mood Disorders

Major Depression

- Major depression is the most severe of depressive disorders.

- Major depression is typically characterized by changes in several areas including mood, behavior, thinking, and physiological processes.

- Specific symptoms of major depression that may be evident include changes in sleep and appetite, changes in physical activity level, loss of energy, feelings of worthlessness, problems with concentration, and thoughts of suicide or actual attempts to commit suicide.

- The frequency of major depression is similar between younger and older individuals.

- Possible causes of major depression include genetic and biological factors, life changes or environmental stresses, and habitual ways of thinking or feeling. Medical problems and certain medications may also cause depression.

- Older people are at greater risk for suicide than younger individuals.

- Treatments for major depression include psychotherapy, medications, and electroconvulsive therapy.

- The majority of older adults can be effectively treated for major depression.

Dysthymia

- This type of depression is less severe than major depression.

- It is a long-standing disturbance of mood in which the individual is depressed most of each day on most days for two years or longer.

- In addition to depressed mood the individual may evidence appetite and sleep problems, tiredness or loss of energy, poor self-esteem, difficulty with concentration, and feelings of hopelessness.

- The frequency of dysthymia in older adults is not well documented, although older adults evidence more individual symptoms of depression than younger adults.

- Treatments include psychotherapy and sometimes medication.

- The effectiveness of treatments for dysthymia in older adults is not well researched. Most older adults, however, appear to respond to treatment.

Bipolar Disorder

- Bipolar disorder was formerly called manic depression.

- People with bipolar disorder have manic episodes in which they may feel especially good, cheerful, "high," or, sometimes, irritable.

- Other possible symptoms of mania include inflated self-esteem, reduced need for sleep, talkativeness, rapid shifting of attention or ideas, easy distractability, increased activity, and involvement in activities that have the potential for serious consequences.

- The vast majority of persons who have episodes of mania also have had major depressive episodes.

- The first episode of mania is usually between the ages of 20 and 40. A manic episode rarely appears for the first time in later life.

- Bipolar disorder affects 1–2% of both the younger and older population.

- Lithium, a psychiatric medication, is the most common treatment for bipolar disorder. Psychotherapy may also be useful in helping people to better contend with life problems caused by bipolar disorder.

- Lithium has been found to be effective in controlling the symptoms of bipolar disorder in the vast majority of younger individuals. It appears to be equally useful in older adults.

Cyclothymia

- A mood disorder that is less severe than bipolar disorder.

- An individual with cyclothymia has periods of hypomania, a less severe form of mania, and periods of depression that are not as severe as major depression.

- Little is known about cyclothymia in older adults.

Introduction

Feelings play a vital role in people's day-to-day lives. The conclusions a person draws about self and world depend, in part, on emotions. If a person is feeling happy, it is more likely that things will look brighter and the individual will engage more vigorously in the world. If feeling depressed, an individual will be more inclined to focus on the negative, the disappointing, and the problematic and to experience less interest in life.

For people of all ages, emotions fluctuate at least somewhat every day. A satisfying visit with a friend of many years may yield a warm emotional glow that lasts through the day. An unexpected disagreement with a spouse may slightly dampen spirits for a few hours or even a few days.

Most individuals have remarked from time to time, "I'm depressed." Though this feeling of being blue, down in the dumps, or sad is unpleasant, it usually passes. For some people, however—young as well as old—feelings of depression do not pass. Days of depression and sadness turn into weeks—and sometimes months. Efforts by loved ones to be helpful and supportive—by being cheerful, offering advice, or taking over responsibilities—have less and less of an effect on the way the person feels.

Occasional feelings of depression—which are part of the texture of our human experience—may become more severe and long lasting. The person may feel trapped in a gloomy emotional existence from which the world looks uninviting and even frightening. Some people who have never experienced prolonged feelings of depression may find themselves in an unfamiliar inner world of emotional darkness. These individuals have what professionals more generally call clinical depression. The word *clinical* simply suggests that the emotional condition is serious enough to warrant help from a mental health professional.

Older individuals are sometimes thought to be "normally" depressed. "After all," people sometimes ask, "wouldn't you be depressed about being old?" The fact is that most older people evidence a significant ability to confront the problems that often accompany aging and still maintain emotional equilibrium. Older adults, like all of us, have days when they feel emotionally out of sorts. Studies suggest, however, that older people have more of these days than younger people. On the other hand, older people do not appear to experience the significant clinical depressions any more frequently than younger adults.

Just as feelings of being sad, blue, or depressed may take hold and make it difficult to experience pleasure or joy, some people have emotional difficulties characterized by feeling too happy, optimistic, or excited. Although this situation is much rarer than depression, people with episodes of what are called mania may experience such strong feelings of enthusiasm and excitement that they make poor judgments about work, their personal lives, or other matters. Almost always, people who have episodes of mania also have periods of depression. Formerly called manic depression, this condition is currently diagnosed as bipolar disorder ("bipolar" in the sense that these individuals experience two different, extreme poles of feeling).

In this chapter on mood disorders major types of clinical depression will be discussed. In the following pages several important questions that older people and their families might ask about depression will be examined:

What is depression?

What causes depression?

How is depression diagnosed by mental health professionals?

How common are different kinds of depression in older adults?

How is depression treated?

How effective are different treatments for depression?

Problems that older people have with the less common disturbance of mood—bipolar disorder and its less serious form, cyclothymia—will also be discussed. As with depression, we will address questions about what these psychiatric problems are, their possible causes, method of diagnosis, frequency among older adults, treatments, and effectiveness of treatments.

Depression

Definition

When an individual complains of being depressed, not caring about things, or having similar feelings, a mental health professional will first be interested in understanding the severity of these feelings and the length of time they have persisted. He or she will also be interested in determining whether the person has also experienced other difficulties that are usually associated with different psychiatric syndromes. A syndrome is a specific group of problems or symptoms that usually occur together. Most psychiatric disorders are syndromes. To make a psychiatric diagnosis, a mental health professional will characterize an individual's problems according to a manual that describes different mental disorders—*The Diagnostic and Statistical Manual of Mental Disorders* (often referred to as *DSM-III-R* because the current version is a revision of the third edition). This manual is periodically revised to take account of new developments in the mental health field. *DSM-III-R* contains specific rules for diagnosing currently recognized mental disorders. The designation and description of mental disorders is based on clinical observation and research. This aggregate of clinical knowledge is important because it informs the mental health professional about the usual causes, complications, and course of the disorder. Although individuals may vary with respect to the symptoms they show, such a classification system allows professionals to meaningfully draw upon the experience of others to develop a plan to provide help to a person with psychiatric problems. A psychiatric diagnosis is a general characterization of a set of problems confronted by an individual. A diagnosis, however, does not tell us who the person is. Competent mental health professionals take into account the unique social, cultural, and psychological characteristics of each individual patient.

The common characteristic of most depressions is the feeling of being sad, downhearted, or blue. Mood is, however, only one feature that characterizes depression. Depression can affect the way a person acts, thinks, and views the world and self. Depression can also significantly alter physiological processes such as sleep and appetite. The pattern, intensity, and duration of depressive symptoms are reviewed by the mental health professional to determine whether an individual has a clinical depression and, if so, what type. Treatment may vary depending on the type of depression. Based on criteria outlined in *DSM-III-R* there are two primary types of clinical depression: major depression and dysthymia.

MAJOR DEPRESSION

Major depression is the most severe of depressive disorders. It is typically characterized by changes in several areas including mood, behavior, thinking, and physiological processes (often referred to as vegetative symptoms) such as sleep and appetite. The presence of only one or a few of these problems does not necessarily indicate a major depression. Although symptoms differ among depressed individuals, some general features lead to a diagnosis of major depression. The following is a summary of the rules outlined in *DSM-III-R* that are used to diagnose a major depressive episode. The full *DSM-III-R* criteria for this and other disorders reviewed in this book may be found in Appendix B.

1. A "dysphoric" mood. These are feelings of being
   depressed, sad, or blue, and/or a significant loss of
   interest or pleasure in life.

2. At least four of the following symptomatic changes have occurred and have lasted a minimum of two weeks:

Changes in appetite. Usually the individual reports loss of appetite sometimes accompanied by weight loss. However, some persons report increased appetite with accompanying weight gain.

Changes in sleep. Typically there will be difficulty in falling asleep (called initial insomnia), staying asleep (middle insomnia), or waking up earlier than usual (terminal insomnia). An individual may experience all or some combination of these types of sleep change. Occasionally, however, individuals complain of sleeping much more than usual.

Psychomotor agitation or retardation. These are clearly observable changes in an individual's physical activity level. Psychomotor agitation is characterized by a tendency to engage in activities such as pacing and wringing of hands. Psychomotor retardation is reflected in an apparent physical slowing down. For example, an individual might get up very slowly from a chair and take much longer to walk to the other side of the room than usual.

Loss of energy. This is the subjective sense that everything is an effort.

Feelings of worthlessness. The individual may have the feeling that he or she is without value or may feel guilty for things he or she did recently or in the past. Sometimes these feelings can be so extreme that they are called delusions—that is, false beliefs that seriously distort reality. For example, a depressed individual may feel that he or she is a source of evil in the world and is being singled out by God for special punishment.

Problems with concentration. Some depressed people may find it very difficult to concentrate, make decisions, or think clearly. An avid newspaper reader, for example, may complain that he is unable to read more than one paragraph without losing attention.

Thoughts of suicide. Suicidal symptoms are ongoing ideas about death or killing oneself that vary in seriousness. Some individuals think, "I'd be better off dead," but would not consider killing themselves. Others make specific plans to kill themselves and are likely to attempt suicide.

3. To be diagnosed with a major depressive episode the individual cannot concurrently have certain other medical or psychiatric problems. These exclusionary conditions include:

An organic condition might be the cause of the depression-related symptoms. Certain physical health problems, for example, are accompanied by depression because they cause physiological imbalances that, when rectified, result in the disappearance of depression.

The depression cannot be part of a usual bereavement reaction to the death of a loved person. In some cases, however, bereavement is so intense and protracted that it subsequently becomes a major depressive episode.

The depression cannot coexist with other specific psychiatric conditions or symptoms. Depressive symptoms can sometimes be part of another psychiatric problem but are not the central feature of the difficulties the individual is experiencing.

4. If a major depressive episode is diagnosed, it is further characterized by its severity (mild, moderate, or severe) and whether it is accompanied by psychotic features. The term *psychotic* refers to a significant distortion of reality such as delusions (false beliefs) or hallucinations (false sensory perceptions). There are various types of delusions and hallucinations, which will be discussed at greater length in Chapter 3.

Delusions or hallucinations sometimes associated with major depression often involve concerns about guilt, death, inadequacy, impoverishment, or punishment. For example, a person might believe he or she is penniless when actually he or she is quite wealthy. An individual experiencing hallucinations might hear voices saying that he or she is a sinner.

Mental health professionals make additional distinctions about a major depressive episode (henceforth referred to as major depression). Major depressions are sometimes classified as chronic (an episode that has lasted at least two years without any significant letup of the depressive symptoms) or recurrent (there have been one or more previous episodes of major depression). The depressive symptoms of some persons are characterized as melancholic. Melancholic depressions are usually more serious than others and accompanied by symptoms that are more biologically determined. Finally, mental health professionals determine whether episodes of major depression occur during certain times of the year, constituting what is called a seasonal pattern.

DYSTHYMIA

Dysthymia is a clinical depression that is less severe than major depression. By definition it is a long-standing disturbance of mood. The following is a summary of *DSM-III-R* rules that define dysthymia.

1. The person has had a depressed mood most of each day on most days for two years or longer. The individual was never without symptoms of depression for more than two months at a time.

2. While depressed, the individual evidences at least two of the following difficulties: appetite changes, sleep problems, tiredness or loss of energy, poor self-esteem, difficulty with concentration or making decisions, and feelings of hopelessness.

3. The above problems are not part of certain other specified psychiatric difficulties.

Dysthymic disorders are also classified according to whether they are related (secondary) or unrelated (primary) to other psychiatric disorders. For example, some persons with alcohol or drug use problems experience depression as a consequence—that is, the depression is a secondary condition of the substance use problem. Dysthymia is also characterized as to whether it appeared early (before age 21) or later in life.

At times it is difficult to distinguish between dysthymia and major depression. Sometimes persons with dysthymia may subsequently, or concomitantly, have an episode of major depression. This has been referred to as a double depression. After the episode of major depression has subsided, they return to their usual selves—that is, they feel chronically depressed.

Although *DSM-III-R*'s descriptions of major depression and dysthymia fairly well characterize most serious depressions, there are other conditions that are accompanied by prominent feelings of depression. Bereavement following the loss of a loved one is a common experience for older adults, with death of a spouse being for the majority of persons their most significant interpersonal loss. Feelings of depression, poor appetite, weight loss, and sleep changes are often part of the "work" of bereavement. These symptoms are seen as normal concomitants of the loss of a significant other and are referred to as uncomplicated bereavement by *DSM-III-R*. Sometimes, however, the grief process does not resolve and the individual may later be regarded as suffering from major depression or dysthymia.

Adjustment disorder is a *DSM-III-R* diagnosis for poor adaptation to a clearly identifiable life stressor or stressors that may involve a depressed mood. In an adjustment disorder, reaction to a stressor either impairs the individual's capacity to function and/or the response to the stress is in excess of what might usually be considered a normal reaction. If the maladaptive response continues six months beyond the onset of the stressor, another diagnosis will usually be assigned. Adjustment disorder is further characterized according to its predominant symptom (e.g., depressed mood, anxious mood, mixed emotional features).

DEPRESSION IN YOUNGER VERSUS OLDER PERSONS

Some researchers have investigated whether the symptoms of depression usually seen in older persons are different from those seen in younger individuals. For the most part, the symptoms are the same although some differences have been noted. Some mental health professionals have reported that older people may be more reluctant to admit to feelings of depression than younger people. Instead they express their emotional distress through physical complaints and symptoms. Physical complaints that have no medical basis and may "mask" an underlying depression have been called depressive equivalents. Some mental health professionals, however, do not accept the notion of masked depression and believe that, with enough time and attention, the usual pattern of symptoms seen in younger people may be elicited from an older person. Diagnosing depression in the aged, however, is sometimes more difficult than in younger individuals. This is because older people often have more physical health problems, take more medications, and, on the whole, experience more isolated symptoms of depression (although not more clinical depression) than younger people. At times, therefore, it is a challenge to determine whether certain possible symptoms of depression are a result of physical illness, medications, or usual stresses of late life. Complex diagnostic issues faced by mental health professionals will be discussed in more detail later in this chapter.

Frequency

Over the years researchers have found it difficult to agree on the frequency (or prevalence) of depression among the aged. In part this is because it was not until 1980 that the psychiatric community developed relatively unambiguous definitions of depressive illness (i.e., the third revision of *The Diagnostic and Statistical Manual of Mental Disorders* was published). Also, some mental health professionals disagree about where to draw the line between normal depression and clinical depression. The distinction between normal and clinical depression is important since older people report much higher rates of depressive symptoms than younger people. Although these individual symptoms in older people generally do not meet stringent *DSM-III-R* criteria for clinical depression, they nevertheless reflect various degrees of emotional suffering. Studies have generally found that about 15 percent of older people living in the community (in distinction from those living in health-related institutions) complain of what is termed significant dysphoria or significant emotional distress. Only 3–4 percent of older people, however, appear to have major depression or dysthymia at any given time. Despite the widely held notion that clinical depression is more common among older adults than younger persons, older adults have similar if not lower rates of depressive illness than do younger age groups.

Some older adults are more vulnerable to depression than others. Among older people with health problems the prevalence of depression is significantly higher than among older people in good health. Some researchers have found that as many as 30–50 percent of older people receiving outpatient medical care have significant depressive symptoms and that those in hospitals may have even higher rates. In long-term care facilities rates of depressive symptoms are also likely to be markedly higher than among community-residing aged. In addition to health problems, other factors are associated with higher rates of depression among the elderly. In both younger and older age groups women are more vulnerable to depression than men. Older persons with lower incomes, less previous education, lower occupational positions, and those who are unmarried (i.e., never-married, divorced, separated, or widowed) are also at greater risk for depression than their peers. As will be discussed later, these factors are probably associated with stress, which increases risk for depression.

Possible Causes

As noted earlier, clinical depression may be associated with changes in many areas of human functioning including feeling, physiology, ways of seeing the world, social interaction, and ability to carry on day-to-day activities. Since clinical depression has such broad effects, researchers have similarly examined a range of possible causes. Current thinking is that clinical depression is probably a function of genetic and biological factors, life changes or environmental stresses, and habitual ways of thinking or acting. For some individuals one of these factors may play the predominant role in precipitating an episode of clinical depression. For many people, however, these factors interact in complex ways to bring about or maintain depression.

GENETICS AND DEPRESSION

Mental health practitioners have long observed that certain kinds of depression are more common in some families than in others. This led researchers to examine whether there might be a genetic component to depression. One problem with trying to investigate this possibility is that there might be reasons other than genetic ones that some families have higher rates of depression than others. For example, certain patterns of child rearing that might predispose persons to depression could be more common in some families. Researchers have found, nevertheless, that some kinds of depression have a clear genetic component. Some of the most convincing evidence comes from research that has examined differences in depression rates between identical (monozygotic) twins and fraternal (dizygotic) twins. Monozygotic twins share exactly the same genetic material while dizygotic twins do not. Between monozygotic twins, we would expect problems with depression in the second twin if the first twin had a history of depression. This pattern should be less likely between dizygotic twins since they share less genetic material. In fact, this has been found to be the case. The same pattern also has been identified among individuals suffering from other kinds of mental disorders such as bipolar disorder and schizophrenia.

It is more likely there is a genetic component to mental disorder when the problem first appears early in life. For example, elderly persons who had their first clinical depressions earlier in life (before age 50) are more likely to have close relatives with depression than those older adults who first became depressed later in life. In recent years there have been many advances in the study of human genetics. We can anticipate a better understanding of the relationship between genetics and mental illness in coming years.

BRAIN CHEMISTRY AND DEPRESSION

Although the phenomenon is not yet well understood, many scientists believe that a genetic predisposition to depression probably reflects differences among people in the production and regulation of certain substances in the brain that may be associated with mood. With the discovery in the 1950s that the drug lithium had a significant and positive effect on mood disorders and the observation that reserpine, a medication for high blood pressure, caused depression in some patients, researchers began to investigate the possible biochemical underpinnings of emotional adjustment. There are several current theories about how brain chemistry affects mood. Interestingly, although antidepressant medications that affect brain chemistry have been clearly shown to help people with clinical depressions, the reasons they work are still the subject of theory and informed speculation.

Information in the brain is communicated by electrical impulses between specialized brain cells called neurons. Electrical impulses cross the gaps between neurons in a several-step process that involves chemical substances called neurotransmitters. Interference or disruption of this delicate process may result in, among other things, poor regulation of mood.

In the catecholamine hypothesis, three substances called amines— norepinephrine, dopamine, and serotonin—are thought to play a major role in the regulation of mood. Norepinephrine, for example, is believed to be released at the gap between two brain neurons. Its release facilitates the transfer of electrical impulses through the brain. After norepinephrine is released, some of it is used again and some of it is deactivated by monoamine oxidase (MAO). Current theories hold that problems in the synthesis of these compounds, the way they are stored, how they are released, and how they are utilized are associated with depression. It is important to note that it is not clear to what extent these hypothesized brain changes are the cause or consequence of depression. For example, a person who underwent a stressful life experience and subsequently became depressed might show the chemical changes predicted by the catecholamine hypothesis. In this case, however, brain chemistry change is most likely not the cause but the effect of depression. Most probably, however, a combination of biological, psychological, and social factors interact to produce and maintain depression.

Why some persons have a first major depression in late life may be puzzling. This is particularly true when the older person confronted significant problems in earlier years, coped with them, and did not become depressed.

Alvin Heller, an affable, robust, 78-year-old man, was being treated with antidepressant medication and was also undergoing individual psychotherapy for a first episode of major depression that had started the previous year. By all objective standards Mr. Heller's later years had been good. His health was fine, his relationship with his wife was seemingly comfortable, and he visited his children often. What was most puzzling was that as a young man Mr. Heller, who was Jewish, had been in a concentration camp, had seen many family members die, and had endured the stresses of immigrating to the United States. Despite these early life experiences, he never became depressed. It was only when he was a relatively old man living under fairly comfortable circumstances that he had a first episode of depression.

Cases like this raise the possibility that aging itself may be associated with brain chemistry changes that predispose some older individuals to depression. Researchers have, in fact, documented increasing amounts of the substance MAO in the brain as people age. This increase might be related to vulnerability to depression in some older persons since, as noted earlier, MAO is thought to deactivate norepinephrine, which appears to play a critical role in mood regulation. Too much MAO might therefore decrease the level of norepinephrine needed for normal mood regulation. Obviously, though, most older people do not get depressed, and increased MAO levels may, for reasons not understood, differentially increase risk for depression. Those who study drug treatments for psychiatric problems—which is called psychopharmacology—are impressed with the variability in people's responses to drugs and to their own emotional vulnerability to environmental stresses. As with the field of genetics, much important work is currently being conducted in the study of the influence of brain structure and biochemistry on mood disorders.

ENVIRONMENTAL STRESSES AND DEPRESSION

Late life is often a time of change. For many persons the relative stability of middle age gives way to life transitions that may or may not have been anticipated. Homemaking and parenting responsibilities wane as children become grown and sometimes move to a different part of the country. People retire or reduce the number of hours they previously devoted to lifelong careers. An acute or chronic physical illness strikes someone who has always been healthy. Researchers who have investigated the effects of stress in younger as well as older people have documented that life changes, particularly undesirable life changes, are associated with physical and mental health problems.

Late-life stresses typically involve the loss of things (e.g., people, money, health) to which the individual has been attached, and loss has been associated with depression. The psychological effects of loss were first studied in children. Researchers found, for example, that children who were separated from their mothers showed behavior that was best characterized as depression. The same was found in studies of infant primates separated from their mothers. The psychological effects of early loss have been found to persist in some persons throughout their lives. For example, adults who, as children, lost one or both parents have a greater risk for depression later in their lives.

Older people have had many years to develop attachments but are also most likely to suffer the loss of the things and people to which they are attached. Attachments are made not only to other persons, but also to places, things, and ideas. In view of the many losses of later life, those who study the elderly have been concerned about the emotional impact of these losses on the aged. As noted, however, while older people are more likely to experience different *symptoms* of depression, they are not more likely to be diagnosed with clinical depression than younger individuals. Despite losses during late life, the majority of older people maintain good emotional equilibrium. Aging may even bring enhanced ability to cope with life stress. Nevertheless, for some older persons, late-life stresses increase the risk for depression.

Usually the most difficult loss is the death of a loved one. Scientists who have tried to quantify the stressfulness of certain life events rate this as one of the most severe. Death of a loved one is usually followed by an expectable period of bereavement. As discussed earlier, bereavement is a normal reaction that is similar to major depression. The length of bereavement varies among individuals and cultural groups. Given the longer life expectancy of women over men, most older women can anticipate grieving the death of their husbands. But many older people also experience the death of friends or acquaintances, which can be very emotionally disconcerting. It has also been recognized that some people form very deep attachments to pets. Some individuals report that the loss of a pet is like the loss of a close friend.

The loss that research studies have most frequently associated with depression is health impairment. The vast majority of elderly people have one or more medical illnesses that sometimes limit their ability to go about their day-to-day lives. In the face of health problems, some individuals feel they have lost a reliable and uncomplaining companion, the body, which now requires regular if not constant attention. For some individuals considerable emotional distress may result from changes in the face or the shape of the body. Acute health problems may leave the individual with a feeling that things have forever changed and that a life with serious physical disabilities is a life not worth living.

> Kurt Weiner, a well-spoken and accomplished man, called the hospital to report that he was bleeding badly from his arm after an "accident." When he arrived at the hospital, he was at first hesitant to explain how he had been hurt. Reluctantly he admitted that he had deliberately cut himself.
>
> A few months prior to the incident Mr. Weiner had experienced a slight stroke that resulted in a mild paralysis of his left arm. Deeply distressed by this, he felt increasingly depressed and hopeless. On the evening that he called the hospital he had became so distressed and angry at his body for "failing" him that he took a kitchen knife and began to hack at his left arm. He was shocked by his own behavior and agreed to accept mental health assistance.

Sociologists, who are concerned with the explicit and implicit rules that govern society, have emphasized the importance of social roles—such as those of worker, spouse, parent, homemaker—as central to the way people define themselves. Social roles are also seen as vehicles for meeting others. One sociologist, Irving Rosow, has argued that the loss of these roles in late life is the largest social challenge that older people face because society generally does not offer new and meaningful roles to replace those that have been lost.

> Pierre LeFort, a 75-year-old former French diplomat, said that he was in distress after his retirement from 35 highly successful years in the foreign service. He admitted that he had never fully realized how much his identity as "the diplomat" defined who he was. He expressed amazement and anger that attempts to set up social engagements with several former associates from the diplomatic corps, whom he considered friends, were cordially turned down. He began to wonder how much his relationships with others had been predicated on his powerful position and considerable influence—and how much they reflected a genuine liking of him as a person.

Loss of a familiar work role at retirement can be very difficult. The fact is, however, that the vast majority of older people retire without significant emotional distress. Clinical experience suggests that those who do have problems have overly defined themselves by their work. Loss of income at retirement may also be stressful for older people. Reduced income not only means fewer resources with which to pursue familiar habits and interests, but also may symbolically be seen as a loss of status.

Finally, there may be the loss of things for which one hoped. Late life may be a time at which one reckons with career goals never reached. It may be a period in which a person realizes that his or her children did not turn out to be the kind of people he or she desired they would be. An individual may be confronted with the reality that he or she did not abide by the ideals he or she felt should have guided his or her life. Or there might be a realization that historical events did not shape the world into a fairer or more peaceful place. Ideas are powerful things and their perceived loss may have emotional repercussions.

PSYCHODYNAMIC APPROACHES TO DEPRESSION

Psychoanalysis and psychodynamic approaches to emotional difficulties go back to early ideas by Sigmund Freud. Freud believed that life involved inherent conflict between the individual's needs and desires and society's demands for conformity to certain ways of behaving. Childhood was seen as the first arena for this conflict, and Freud placed emphasis on early childhood experiences as critical determinants of later psychological development. An individual's personality, in part, he believed, reflected the characteristic manner in which the tension between one's needs and the demands of the world was managed. Freud's ideas have been refined, expanded, and challenged by succeeding generations of psychodynamically oriented mental health professionals. Some strictly adhere to Freud's and his early followers' ideas. Others regard these precepts as thoughtful insights into the human condition but believe they fall far short of fully portraying the nature of human psychology. It was Freud and his followers who questioned the usefulness of psychological treatments for older people since the aged were presumed to be too "rigid" to change.

From a psychodynamic perspective, long-standing depression in an individual may be seen as reflecting underlying conflicts not directly conscious to the person. These conflicts may be too painful for the person to consciously recognize but may nevertheless exert a negative influence on the individual's life. Emotional difficulties such as depression may appear for no apparent reason. Psychodynamically oriented mental health professionals search to determine the possible causes. For example, a previously active, independent individual may experience serious depression in later life over issues of increasing dependency on others. This person may have had early conflicts over dependency on his parents that have special meaning. Psychodynamic theories hold that the understanding and experience of the underlying conflict will result in reduced depression and improvement in daily life.

COGNITIVE AND BEHAVIORAL
APPROACHES TO DEPRESSION

Some theories of depression place critical importance on the emotional consequences of the characteristic manner in which people act and think. Behaviorally oriented psychologists believe that people's behavior is strongly influenced by the rewards, lack of rewards, or punishments that precede and follow the behavior. For example, if an individual has spent a gratifying time with another person, it is more likely that he or she will make additional plans to see that person. One well-known behavioral approach suggests that depression may begin when the individual starts to reduce the frequency of doing things that have usually brought praise, concern, or the like from others—in the parlance of behaviorists, these things are reinforcements. One possible reason for a change in behavior may be that significant others fail to provide the usual level of responsiveness to the individual's behavior and, as a result, the frequency of that behavior decreases. To continue the above example, if visits to a friend are found increasingly unsatisfying, it is less likely that the friend will be visited as frequently. There may also be major changes in the availability of a person or persons on whom the individual depends for gratification. If a lifelong friend with whom a person organized his or her social life dies, the individual may not feel like going out as often and may experience the feeling that life is just not the same without that friend.

Two others factors play a part in behavioral formulations about depression. Once depressed, an individual may be inadvertently rewarded or reinforced for the depressive behavior. Although this may sound counterintuitive, in clinical practice it is sometimes seen. Depressed persons, who complain about the way they feel or the things that trouble them, at first receive sympathetic concern and attention. This attention may actually reward the depressive behavior, which—in theory—will therefore be more likely to persist. As time goes on, other individuals will eventually tire of the complaints and aversive behavior shown by the depressed person. Interactions with the depressed person become less enjoyable and others may find themselves wanting to spend less time with him or her. The depressed individual may make even louder or more dramatic complaints in order to get the previous level of attention, which, in turn, may further reinforce the depressive behavior. The depressed person may also eventually turn to people who were previously unfamiliar with his or her depression difficulties. At first, these people will respond with the usual expressions of concern. Depression may also be reinforced by the fact that it provides a socially acceptable reason for relief from unpleasant life responsibilities (for example, housework).

Another behavioral perspective suggests that individuals who initially possess fewer social skills may be most vulnerable to depression. Such individuals may be especially sensitive to the exit of friends from their lives (for example, because of death or moving) and may not be able to develop new friendships.

Another major psychological approach to depression was initially developed by psychiatrist Aaron Beck. Dr. Beck posited that an important component of and risk factor for depression is the way the individual looks at self and world. Beck identified what he calls the cognitive triad of negative thoughts—related to oneself, one's current experiences, and the future. The depressed or depression-prone individual has the tendency to view things in a characteristically negative manner. The longer-range impact of such a negatively skewed point of view is depression. Depressed mood itself then inclines the individual to think even more negatively about him- or herself and current and future circumstances, creating a vicious cycle of negative thinking and negative mood. Imagine the emotional impact on yourself of spending an hour thinking about every past life failure and every imaginable problem that might befall you in the next several years. At the end of the hour your mood would probably be distressed, anxious, or depressed. Some depressed individuals spend months in this mental process.

Essentially, Beck and his colleagues argue that patterns of thinking play an important mediating role between what happens on a day-to-day basis and mood. They also argue that thinking patterns are amenable to change by experienced cognitive therapists. Some cognitive theorists assert that persons vulnerable to depression have an ongoing tendency to view the world in rigid and negative ways. Although there is research evidence that demonstrates that, when depressed, people do indeed tend to see things in negative ways, there is not strong evidence that depressed people held such views more often than other people before becoming depressed.

> Frances Warton came to the clinic at the behest of
> her family, who were deeply distressed at the changes
> that had come over her in the last year. In their view
> Frances had gone from being a pleasant, outgoing,
> socially active, "upbeat" person to a withdrawn and
> particularly negative individual. "She's not the same
> person," they lamented.

Frances reluctantly began to talk about what had happened in her recent life. "What's the use? Nothing will help. My life is over," she repeated over and over at first. Frances reported that retirement was especially hard for her and that it had been compounded by the diagnosis of a chronic medical problem that was disfiguring her. Over time, she withdrew from others and stopped doing the things she most enjoyed because of concerns about the way she looked. "Frankly, Doctor, I'm useless and hopeless and I don't know why you're wasting your time on someone like me."

Evaluation

A thorough diagnostic evaluation of an older person suspected of having a clinical depression is the first critical step in obtaining mental health assistance. The diagnostic skills of the mental health professional may literally have life and death ramifications for the older adult. The fact is that diagnosing mental health problems in older people is usually more difficult than in younger persons. This is because many older people experience a variety of medical illnesses, take medications, and confront an array of late-life stresses that may or may not be relevant to the apparent clinical depression. Mental health professionals, of course, differ in their preferred styles of doing a diagnostic work-up. Unfortunately, they may also vary in their knowledge of age-related issues and their competence to adequately assess those issues. The following describes what is generally considered a good work-up—good in the sense that it covers the psychiatric, psychological, social, cultural, and medical factors currently believed to be relevant to clinical depression.

ESTABLISHING A GOOD RAPPORT WITH THE OLDER PERSON

Older people are not usually enthusiastic about being brought for a mental health evaluation. Particularly for people of the current older generation, seeing a mental health professional has negative implications and, for some, may be seen as a threatening or humiliating experience. If the older individual is indeed depressed, the situation is compounded by the tendency of depressed persons to focus on the negative and view things as hopeless.

It is often family members who have urged the older person to come for an evaluation. Family members have also usually done considerable advance work prior to the first evaluation. This has included locating a presumably competent mental health professional, consulting with other family members, and trying to persuade the older person to actually go for the evaluation. Family members of course vary in their capacity to skillfully arrange for a first evaluation.

> Rose Gibson was sitting quietly by her daughter in the clinic waiting room when the psychiatrist introduced herself and invited Mrs. Gibson to come to her office. Mrs. Gibson looked puzzled and then panicked. Reluctantly she accompanied the psychiatrist to her office. Mrs. Gibson did not understand why the psychiatrist was asking her so many "personal" questions. Eventually it was learned that Mrs. Gibson's daughter had told her that she was being taken to a senior citizens center where she would take part in "activities." Later Mrs. Gibson's daughter said she did this because, "My mother would never have come if she knew I was taking her to a psychiatrist." Mrs. Gibson refused to return for a follow-up visit.

Even if family members have done a good job of explaining why they want the older person to undergo an evaluation, it is useful for the mental health professional to make sure that at the outset the purpose of the visit is clear.

Adjustments must sometimes be made for perceptual or intellectual limitations of the older person. It is important from the beginning for the mental health professional to learn whether the older person has hearing problems and, if so, which is the "best side" to which conversation should be directed. Some older people with hearing problems will smile pleasantly and nod without understanding what is being said to them. Use of nontechnical language is also important so that questions are communicated unambiguously. If the older person does need treatment, the likelihood of a return visit will, in part, depend on this initial mental health contact. Particularly with older people, it is useful to get additional information from other family members — the spouse and/or adult children can often be helpful. This may be done after an initial interview with the older person.

EVALUATION OF CURRENT PROBLEMS

As was discussed earlier in this chapter, a psychiatric diagnosis is made on the basis of rules outlined in *The Diagnostic and Statistical Manual of Mental Disorders* (*DSM-III-R*) of the American Psychiatric Association. In making a psychiatric diagnosis it is important to know the nature of current problems, their severity, how long they have existed, how they may have changed over time, to what degree they impair the person's usual level of activity or functioning, and whether their onset coincided with other problems or changes. For example, an older adult might state that she has felt depressed, guilty, and uninterested in things. These symptoms have been accompanied by poor appetite and sleeping difficulties for the past three months and the condition is so bad the individual reports, "I can't stand it." Further, these problems started after the death of her best friend, whom she had known since childhood. She also reports that she has seen many fewer people than usual and that she has increasingly fallen behind with her housework. It is usual in a diagnostic interview to inquire whether the person may be experiencing other types of difficulties (for example, hallucinations or delusions) or problems with cognitive functioning (for example, problems with memory, attention, the ability to abstract ideas) and whether the individual has had any suicidal or homicidal ideas or plans.

As noted earlier, some research has found that a few characteristics of clinical depression may differ between older and younger people. Mental health professionals report that some older patients will complain of physical symptoms instead of feelings of depression even when depression exists. These complaints have been called depressive equivalents that mask depression. Some depressive equivalents that have been noted include pain (especially in the back, neck, or head), gastrointestinal symptoms (for example, constipation or fleeting abdominal distress), and discomfort in the mouth. The notion of masked depression or depressive equivalents is, however, the subject of some disagreement among geriatric mental health professionals. Some argue that careful evaluation will elicit reports of the usual symptoms of depression from older patients who, at first, only focus on physical symptoms. Of course, physical complaints by an older person should be taken seriously since they may signal the presence of bona fide medical problems.

EVALUATION OF PAST PROBLEMS

To best understand current depression problems it is important to understand any previous problems. Some older people have had lifelong difficulties with depression. For others, the current problems are the first time they have ever experienced significant mental health difficulties. Inquiries should be made by a mental health professional about whether the individual has a history of other major psychiatric difficulties—for example, a history of alcohol or drug dependence.

DETERMINATION OF MEDICAL PROBLEMS

A vague general inquiry about the older person's physical health is not adequate. The symptoms usually seen in clinical depression may be signaling the presence of a serious medical problem that has not been diagnosed. These symptoms may also be the direct result of certain medications or combinations of medications. With the help of family members, a past and current medical history should be compiled by an individual with medical training.

Depression is sometimes one of many symptoms associated with some medical illnesses. For example, the incidence of depression among people suffering from Parkinson's disease (a neurological disorder characterized by difficulties in moving, muscular rigidity, and shaking) is quite high (estimates range from 40–90 percent). Other medical conditions that may be associated with depression are thyroid disease (a disorder of the endocrine system), cancer of the pancreas, viral infections, high blood pressure, strokes, heart problems, gastrointestinal problems, and genitourinary dysfunction (difficulties with urination or defecation).

If, at the time of evaluation for depression, the older adult has not had a recent physical examination, one should be done. A medical evaluation usually includes a general physical; neurological, pelvic, and rectal exams; blood pressure readings; an electrocardiogram or EKG (which measures heart activity); and blood tests, urinalysis, thyroid tests, and other specialized tests that may be needed. A clear understanding of the older person's medical history is also important if a psychiatrist intends to prescribe psychotropic (psychiatric) medications. Some medications may aggravate coexisting medical conditions. For example, tricyclic antidepressants must be used cautiously in persons with a history of heart problems.

MEDICATION AS A CAUSE OF DEPRESSION

Some geriatric psychiatrists have noted, "If a medication can help, it can also hurt." Medications are powerful compounds that have both intended and unintended effects. Prescribing a medication typically involves a trade-off between its ability to alleviate or improve existing problems and its undesired side effects.

Many older people take a lot of medications. An average older person fills 13 prescriptions a year; people 65 or older order almost three times as many prescriptions as persons younger than 65. There are potential dangers for older persons taking several medications at the same time. Most people, whether young or old, generally do not comply well with directions given to them by physicians on how to take medications. Compliance with medication directions may be particularly difficult for older people with visual or memory problems and may be enormously complicated for those taking multiple pills at several different times each day.

Sometimes a physician fails to adequately inquire or older persons fail to inform the physician about medications that are being taken. As previously noted, some medications are known to cause depression. Some combinations of medications may lead to symptoms that mimic certain psychiatric difficulties. In addition to prescribed medications, some older people may be taking over-the-counter remedies that, when mixed with prescribed medication, cause problems. Given the large number of possible combinations of medications that might be taken at any one time, the effect of some drug combinations is not known. Nevertheless, all suspected drug side effects should be evaluated by a physician.

Certain high blood pressure medications (most notably, reserpine) and some psychiatric medications (for example, anti-psychotic or anti-anxiety drugs) may cause depression. In addition, some medications for sleep problems (hypnotics), pain (narcotics), or allergies (antihistamines) can prompt depressive symptoms. The effects from these drugs may be subtle and not readily noticeable. For example, an older person may complain of tiredness and a lack of interest in life. An astute psychiatrist might hypothesize that these changes are medication effects. In conjunction with the physician who is prescribing a medication, the psychiatrist might temporarily decrease or discontinue a medication(s). A less astute health professional, however, might consider these symptoms signs of aging.

THE PERSONAL, SOCIAL, AND CULTURAL CONTEXTS OF LATE-LIFE DEPRESSION

Dr. Robert Butler, a geriatric psychiatrist and the first director of the National Institute on Aging, has argued that a psychiatric diagnosis is a critical step in the mental health evaluation of an older person. He emphasizes, however, that it is only one of the steps. An older individual, for example, may clearly meet the *DSM-III-R* criteria for major depression, but a variety of other factors may be central to understanding why the individual became depressed and has stayed depressed and to deciding which psychotherapeutic or psychopharmacologic treatments may be most appropriate.

An older individual who walks into the mental health professional's office possesses six or more decades of experiences that have been sculpted by unique generational events (for example, the Great Depression and World War II), outlooks influenced by race or culture, political beliefs, philosophical or religious ideas, and characteristic patterns of interacting with relatives and friends. One or more of these factors may bear on why the person came for an evaluation in the first place—and on whether the offer of mental health assistance will be accepted. The mental health professional's failure to familiarize him- or herself with the personal and interpersonal landscape of the older person can impair attempts to seriously engage the individual in a treatment plan that is realistic.

Dr. Butler and his associates have developed a personal data form that they use to evaluate a broad range of past and current life issues that may bear on the older person's current problems.

Dr. Butler likens the personal data form to a psychosocial electro-cardiogram. The following areas are reviewed with the older person: basic background information; religious affiliation/influences; past and current family status (e.g., marriages, children, grandchildren); early family history; education; work history; retirement experience; economic resources; current residential arrangements; transportation and physical mobility status; interests/sources of pleasure; community involvement; patterns of friendship; experience with social prejudice; attitudes toward death and dying; thoughts about past and current self; and a detailed review of medical, psychiatric, and medication history. In the process of gathering this information, rapport can often be developed by discussing problems and prospects and successes and sorrows of the older person.

SUICIDE, DEPRESSION, AND OLDER PEOPLE

It comes as a surprise to most people to learn that the highest rate of suicide is among the white elderly population. On average, 25 percent of suicides in the United States each year are committed by older people—even though they make up about 11 percent of the population. Among older adults, white men are most at risk for suicide. The reasons for the high suicide rate among elderly men have not been carefully explored. It has been suggested that in this society white men stand to lose more power, status, and influence in their later years than do either women or nonwhite men. The losses of late life may come as a shock to some older white men who may not have adequately developed personal identities and coping capabilities apart from those specific to the workplace. The loss of functional capacities that occurs with some physical illnesses may represent to some older men an unacceptable loss of control over their destinies. This may precipitate depression and suicidal feelings. The case of Kurt Weiner, discussed earlier, is probably an example of this kind of problem in adapting to late life.

The reasons older people try to commit or succeed at committing suicide are varied, but physical illness may be the most important factor. Other risk factors include previous suicide attempts, alcohol use, divorce, and widowhood. It appears that while the majority of older persons who commit suicide are probably significantly depressed (estimates range from 50–80 percent), some persons who kill themselves are not seriously depressed.

When older people attempt suicide, they are often successful. The best estimates are that 1 out of 4 suicide attempts by older people are successful. This is in contrast to 1 out of 20 successful attempts in persons younger than 40. Also in contrast to younger people, older people are more likely to complete the act of suicide rather than to threaten suicide. Some individuals may slowly kill themselves by deliberately neglecting nutrition and medication.

Any expression of suicidal thoughts by an older person must be taken seriously. Careful inquiries need to be made. Suicidal tendencies vary on a continuum from vague, occasional thoughts like "I might be better off dead" to a well thought out suicide plan that the individual intends to carry out. In general, the more detailed the person's thinking about how a suicide would be carried out, the greater should be the family's and the mental health professional's concern. Sometimes, however, there is no clear warning.

Thomas Franklin was a handsome, very independent 77-year-old man. A widower, he lived alone and was for the most part socially isolated. He had come to the outpatient geriatric mental health clinic from a psychiatric inpatient service where he had been treated for a major depression that was accompanied by suicidal thoughts.

Despite a year of tricyclic antidepressant pharmacotherapy and supportive psychotherapy, Mr. Franklin remained mildly to moderately depressed. He nevertheless continued to drive his automobile, which enabled him to occasionally see former work acquaintances, run errands, and attend medical and mental health appointments. One day he arrived at his weekly psychotherapy appointment by taxi cab instead of by car. He explained that he could no longer drive his car because he had lost the vision in his right eye. A call to his physician revealed that, indeed, he had had a hemorrhage that left him blind in one eye with the possibility of the total loss of sight in his other eye. In the next week's psychotherapy session, Mr. Franklin said that he would be feeling "pretty good" if it were not for his eye. He described himself as "annoyed" by his medical condition but denied serious depressive feelings or suicidal concerns.

Mr. Franklin did not show up for his next appointment. After repeated attempts were made to contact him by telephone, a call was made to a neighbor, who said that Mr. Franklin had committed suicide the previous week. Later it was learned that he took an overdose of antidepressants and left a note saying that he felt his life was not worth living in view of failing eyesight and inability to drive his car.

COGNITIVE CHANGES AND DEPRESSION

In the 1950s psychiatrists Sir Martin Roth and Dr. Felix Post conducted research that challenged an assumption held by most medical professionals at that time. The assumption was that cognitive and emotional problems seen in older people were part of a common process of degeneration of the brain. Drs. Roth and Post carefully evaluated older persons with different kinds of psychiatric problems and later evaluated these individuals again to determine the outcome of their difficulties. Roth and Post found that the significant cognitive changes consistent with a diagnosis of dementia and the emotional difficulties characterized by depression were, in fact, two different kinds of diseases that had very different outcomes. Older people with dementia got worse while the condition of depressed older people generally improved.

Depressed persons, however, sometimes evidence changes—notably concentration difficulties, memory complaints, and poor judgment—that can be mistaken for dementia. Given the greatly different outcomes of dementia and clinical depression, an error in diagnosis may have terrible consequences. There are cases, for example, of persons with severe depressions who were thought to have dementia and therefore were not treated but instead were placed in nursing homes, where they gradually deteriorated.

The presence of significant cognitive changes in depressed older people has been called pseudodementia. The term primarily describes cognitive changes that, on successful treatment of a mental health problem like depression, are no longer evident. Some have objected to the use of the term *pseudodementia* and prefer somewhat more descriptive labels like "reversible dementia caused by depression." Pseudodementia is not a formal diagnostic term used by *DSM-III-R*. Rather it is a caveat to mental health professionals that they must carefully evaluate both the psychiatric and cognitive status of individuals who present a mix of mental changes. It is important to note, however, that individuals whose primary problem is dementia may also be depressed. These issues are discussed in Chapter 3.

Treatment

Until recently, many health professionals and the public alike tended to regard old age as an inevitable period of mental and emotional decline about which little could be done. Depression in late life was seen as an expectable response to circumstances that would just have to be endured. Sigmund Freud helped to set the stage for the pessimism about the utility of mental health services for older adults when he expressed considerable doubt about the ability of older people to change. Older people were seen by Freud as not possessing the necessary energy to confront the underlying psychological conflicts that were thought to cause emotional misery. There are a variety of somatic (drug and electroconvulsive therapies) and psychological (individual, marital, family, and group psychotherapies) interventions that have been developed for younger persons and are increasingly being utilized with older individuals. The fact is, however, that most research on somatic and psychological interventions for depression have not explored whether response to these treatments differs according to age. Many studies of the efficacy of certain antidepressants, for example, have systematically excluded people 65 years or older. This is usually because older people often have one or more medical problems that can complicate the interpretation of research findings. It is easier to conduct studies with medically healthy younger persons. We therefore have less information on which treatments might be most effective for the elderly. Nevertheless, it appears that most major treatments offered to younger persons are usually effective in older persons if they are modified to take into account the specific social, psychological, and biological changes associated with getting older. Fortunately, in the last few years the pace of research on somatic psychotherapeutic treatments for depressed older people has quickened.

In the following section, we will examine the usual somatic and psychological treatments that are offered to people with clinical depression, with special interest in how these treatments need to be modified for the elderly.

SOMATIC TREATMENTS

In the last 25 years there have been major advances in the pharmacological (psychiatric drug) treatment of depression. A variety of compounds have been proven to hasten the end of episodes of depression and to reduce the frequency of their recurrence. Most notably, tricyclic antidepressants (*tricyclic* refers to the characteristic molecular make-up of a common type of antidepressant) have been widely prescribed by medical and psychiatric care practitioners. Electroconvulsive therapy (colloquially, and incorrectly, referred to as shock therapy) has been used for many years and continues to be used under certain circumstances.

Unfortunately, psychotropic medications have not always been prescribed wisely to the elderly. These medications may not only have favorable effects on older people's depression, but may also have potent side effects, some of which may be life threatening. Prescribing psychotropic medications such as antidepressants requires a basic understanding by the psychiatrist of the biological differences between older and younger people. We will review some of these basic issues before discussing the usual kinds of somatic treatments for depression.

How Drugs Are Utilized in the Human Body

When taking a medication most of us give little thought to what happens once it enters the body. Our main interest is that the medication relieves or eliminates the symptoms that concern us or our physician. Utilization of medication by the body is a complex and dynamic process. As people age, the manner in which they process medications changes. A medical doctor's failure to reckon with those changes may result in an inability of the aging body to make full use of the therapeutic potential of a drug—or may even result in serious harm to the older individual.

The purpose of most psychotropic drugs is to change certain aspects of brain chemistry thought to cause the psychiatric problem. With depression, for example, antidepressants are believed to increase the amount of substances called biogenic amines (like norepinephrine) in the brain. This is thought to help alleviate symptoms of depression. The process of drug disposition—from the point the drug is ingested, gets to the brain, and then is metabolized or broken down—is referred to as pharmacokinetics. The pharmacokinetic aspects of psychotropic drugs in late life have only recently been the focus of research, some of which has helped to better explain, for example, why older people typically need smaller amounts of drugs and are often more sensitive to the side effects of psychiatric medications than younger people are.

There are three central concepts in pharmacokinetics: absorption (how the drug gets into the system), distribution (how the drug is dispersed throughout the body), and elimination (how the drug is eventually eliminated from the body).

Most drugs are typically taken orally by the older person and are absorbed in the gastrointestinal tract (the stomach and intestines). The rate at which the gastrointestinal tract acts upon the drug will determine how long the drug takes to get into the system. Although there are some age-related changes in this process, on the whole these changes do not appear to significantly affect absorption.

Once a drug has been absorbed, it begins to be dispersed throughout the body. Drugs are stored in certain areas of the body. For example, most antidepressants are stored in fatty tissues. Therefore the amount and proportion of fat in a particular person's body will affect how much of a drug is stored. This issue is particularly important for older people because they (most notably women) typically have a much higher proportion of body fat (compared with muscle) than younger people do. This means that older people store larger amounts of antidepressants in their bodies and that, in turn, it takes longer for the drugs to be eliminated from their systems. Another issue is that once a drug has entered the circulatory system, some of the drug attaches itself to certain substances in the blood (most notably plasma albumin). Some drugs do this more than others. That part of the drug that does *not* attach is available to do the intended pharmacological work. In the aged, however, there are usually lower levels of plasma albumin to which a drug can attach. Therefore older people may have more "unbound" drug (drug that can exert the intended effect) than younger people given the same dosage.

Most drugs are eliminated through two major organ systems: the liver and the kidneys. When blood containing the drug passes through the liver, most of the drug is removed and subjected to chemical changes involving certain enzymes, which begin to deactivate the drug. In older people, the liver does not typically work as efficiently as in younger people. The final stage of elimination is in the kidneys. Like the liver, the kidneys work less efficiently in older adults than in younger persons, and it usually takes longer to eliminate most drugs from the system.

The practical implication of the above factors is that older people typically need smaller doses of medication, tend to be more sensitive to the side effects of drugs, and take longer to eliminate drugs from their systems. A related and often complex issue is the interaction of different psychiatric medications with medical medications. The usefulness of some antidepressants can be greatly reduced if, for example, the individual is receiving some types of high blood pressure medications. The presence of certain medical illnesses can also affect the way in which the body processes and utilizes pharmaceuticals.

Medication Treatment of Depression in the Elderly

The decision to prescribe psychotropic medications to a depressed older person is based on several factors including physical health, kinds of depression symptoms, previous response to psychotropic medications, and social and psychological characteristics of the older person that might bear on ability to take medications properly. Some mental health professionals feel that antidepressant medications are too readily prescribed to older people who may need, instead of or in addition to the medication, an opportunity to sort out complex life problems in psychotherapy. Others argue, however, that since only a small fraction of depressed older people actually get treatment, all forms of mental health assistance, including antidepressant treatment, need to be made more widely available. The fact is that antidepressant treatment can significantly alleviate depression in the majority of older persons when prescribed by competent medical professionals who are aware of basic issues in the biology, psychology, and sociology of aging.

Three basic types of drugs are used to treat depression: tricyclic antidepressants, monoamine oxidase (MAO) inhibitors, and so-called second-generation antidepressants. Persons with bipolar disorder are also usually treated with the drug lithium. Sometimes other medications (lithium or the thyroid replacement T3) are added to antidepressants. The generic and trade names of the most common antidepressants and other psychotropic medications may be found in Appendix A.

TRICYCLIC ANTIDEPRESSANTS   Tricyclic antidepressants are often prescribed for individuals with major depression. As noted earlier, major depressions are usually accompanied by problems with sleep, appetite, and energy that are thought to be caused by changes in brain chemistry. It is generally believed that people with major depression are the best candidates for antidepressants. More recently, however, there has been increasing interest in prescribing antidepressants for people with dysthymia.

If a psychiatrist is considering using an antidepressant medication, a knowledge of the medical condition of the patient is critical. In addition to providing a complete history of current and past medical problems, the patient should undergo certain medical tests that help to rule out other explanations for depression-related symptoms. Some medical tests are also used to determine whether the individual has a medical condition that may preclude the use of antidepressants. Most notably, some people with heart problems cannot be prescribed antidepressants because the medication may seriously aggravate the existing heart condition.

There are two primary kinds of tricyclic antidepressants: tertiary amines and secondary amines. The names refer to the chemical structure of the drugs. There have been numerous studies to determine which tricyclic antidepressant(s) may be most effective. On the whole, these antidepressants have been shown to be equally effective. The choice of an antidepressant usually depends on: (1) the type and severity of side effects typically associated with a particular antidepressant and, if applicable, (2) the individual's previous response to an antidepressant. While no single antidepressant has been found to be generally superior, some individuals respond much better to one type of antidepressant than to another. This reflects the usual variability in people's physiological make-up.

For elderly persons the "side-effect profile" of an antidepressant may play a critical role in its choice. As discussed, because of biological changes associated with aging, older people are usually more sensitive to the side effects of drugs. Some side effects may be desirable. For example, a very agitated depressed person may benefit from a drug that has a sedating effect. For the most part, however, most psychiatrists want to minimize side effects.

Tricyclic antidepressants have several major types of side effects. These include cardiac changes, blood pressure changes, sedation, and what are called anticholinergic effects. Each of these will be discussed.

Cardiac changes are a type of antidepressant side effect that should be of most concern to a psychiatrist prescribing these drugs. A variety of cardiac difficulties, some of them potentially life threatening, have been associated with use of antidepressants. For most persons with current or previous heart conditions a careful determination must be made whether antidepressants should be prescribed. Examples of these heart conditions are bundle branch disease, heart block, cardiac arrhythmias, congestive heart failure, and past history of myocardial infarction. If antidepressants are prescribed, the cardiac condition of the patient must be closely monitored. Those persons most at risk for cardiac side effects from these medications are those with past or current heart problems; for the most part, persons without heart problems are much less likely to experience cardiac-related side effects.

The second most serious side effect of tricyclic antidepressants is a condition called orthostatic hypotension. This is a sudden drop of blood pressure that occurs particularly when an individual sits up or stands up quickly. The greatest danger is that the person may fall. Especially with the elderly, there is risk of bone fractures from falling. Older adults should be cautioned that when taking antidepressants they should stand up slowly. One good way to evaluate the likelihood of orthostatic change is to take an individual's blood pressure both while he or she is sitting and while he or she is standing before starting the medication, and then to continue to monitor the patient's blood pressure throughout drug treatment. Differences between blood pressure while seated and blood pressure while standing give an indication of the degree to which orthostatic hypotension may be a problem.

Another side effect of antidepressants is sedation. Drugs differ in the extent to which they sedate and, as noted, sedation may initially be desired for a person who has agitated depression or has marked problems with sleep. Once the individual is feeling better, however, less sedation is typically desired. Since drugs generally remain longer in older people's systems than in those of younger adults, older people may complain of sleepiness during the day. For this reason, some psychiatrists recommend tricyclic antidepressants for the elderly that are less sedating.

The most common type of side effect from antidepressants is that classified as anticholinergic. Cholinergic functions are involved in many bodily systems; anticholinergic side effects, by definition, are the results of interference with normal cholinergic functioning by antidepressants. Patients may experience a dry mouth and/or constipation due to antidepressants. For a dry mouth, physicians will often recommend chewing gum or eating sugarless candies to aid in lubrication of the mouth. In the case of constipation, dietary changes or bulk laxative are sometimes recommended. Other anticholinergic side effects include urinary retention (difficulties with urination), exacerbation of prostatic hypertrophy (worsening of prostate problems in men), and potential worsening of glaucoma. These difficulties can usually be managed successfully by carefully adjusting the patient's medication. These side effects may also lessen in severity over time.

Of the two primary classes of tricyclic antidepressants, tertiary amines and secondary amines, secondary amines are usually more frequently recommended for the elderly. This is because tertiary amines are processed by the body in a more complicated fashion and, on the whole, tend to have more side effects than secondary amines. As with most drugs, psychotropic medications have both generic (scientific) and trade (commercial) names. This multiplicity of names for the same drug sometimes leads to confusion for older patients and their families. When starting one of these medications with an older person, the psychiatrist will usually begin with a dosage considerably smaller than what will be the final target dose. This is done so that the individual's body may gradually accommodate to the drug. With larger initial doses the individual would probably experience strong side effects. As the psychiatrist slowly increases the medication, he or she will evaluate the kind and severity of side effects the patient may be experiencing. Often within three to four weeks some improvement in the depression will be seen, although responses vary. If the individual is going to improve on the antidepressant, progress should usually be seen within six weeks. Sometimes patients do not improve within this period of time and the psychiatrist may change the medication to see if another type of antidepressant is more effective.

There has been considerable discussion among psychiatrists in recent years about the importance of keeping people on antidepressants long enough and at high enough doses to ensure that the medication actually will work. Some psychiatrists may prematurely conclude that a particular medication is not useful when actually the patient is simply not getting enough of it. Sometimes a blood test is taken to measure the actual amount of antidepressant in the blood. A given individual may seem to be getting an adequate dose of medication, yet, because of the particular way his or her system processes the antidepressant, only a small amount can be detected in the blood. In this case, a psychiatrist may choose to increase the dosage.

Another reason that older people in particular may be prematurely discontinued from an antidepressant is side effects. It may take considerable patience on the part of both the older person and the psychiatrist to manage unpleasant side effects. It may mean, for example, increasing the dosage much more slowly than usual. Side effects are frequently less severe this way.

As noted earlier, after careful assessment of the older person's response to a particular antidepressant, the psychiatrist may choose to prescribe another. Some psychiatrists will try another tricyclic antidepressant while others will use a different class of antidepressants called MAO inhibitors.

MONOAMINE OXIDASE (MAO) INHIBITORS   While it is thought that tricyclic antidepressants increase the amount of norepinephrine in the brain, MAO inhibitors reduce the activity of MAO—a substance that metabolizes (biologically breaks down) norepinephrine. By inhibiting the breakdown of norepinephrine, more of it should be available in the brain; in theory, this will reduce depression symptoms. As mentioned, MAO levels increase with age—which may predispose some older people to depression in later life.

The major drawback of MAO inhibitors is that they require a restricted diet because of the possibility of a hypertensive crisis. The substance tyramine, found in a variety of foods (for example, cheese, sausage, beef, and chicken liver), may interact with MAO inhibitors to significantly increase blood pressure and with it the risk for stroke. Other drugs may also interact with MAO inhibitors with the same effect. Some geriatric psychiatrists believe that, for the most part, MAO inhibitors should not be prescribed for the elderly. Others have found that these medications can significantly improve depression in older people and may be used safely. Almost all agree, however, that unless an older person can reliably follow a restricted diet, he or she should not be prescribed MAO inhibitors.

Some persons taking MAO inhibitors gain a great deal of weight. Others report sexual problems, most notably difficulty in reaching orgasm. Some men taking MAO inhibitors have difficulty achieving an erection. Like tricyclic antidepressants, MAO inhibitors may also cause orthostatic hypotension, anticholinergic-like effects (dry mouth, constipation, urinary retention), and sedation. MAO inhibitors should be initially prescribed in small doses and the dosage should be increased slowly. They should also be prescribed for a long enough period of time so that the psychiatrist can determine their efficacy.

Both tricyclic antidepressants and MAO inhibitors may be prescribed for varying lengths of time. For an individual with a first serious episode of depression, the medication is often prescribed for about six months, gradually reduced, and then stopped. For a person who has had two or more episodes of serious depression, antidepressant medication may be prescribed on an ongoing basis. The reason for chronic treatment is to reduce the likelihood of future episodes.

ATYPICAL "SECOND-GENERATION" ANTIDEPRESSANTS   A more recently developed group of antidepressant medications, sometimes referred to as second-generation antidepressants, have a chemical structure that is different from tricyclics or MAO inhibitors. Examples of these include trazodone (trade name Desyrel), fluoxetine (Prozac), bupropion (Wellbutrin), and amoxapine (Ascendin). Some of the medications are believed to operate more selectively on the biochemical systems involved in depression than do tricyclics or MAO inhibitors. Some of these medications do not have the side effects usually associated with tricyclics or MAO inhibitors but, unfortunately, may have other side effects. Most of these compounds have not been carefully studied in the elderly although they are prescribed for this age group.

OTHER MEDICATIONS SOMETIMES PRESCRIBED WITH ANTIDEPRESSANTS
After a psychiatrist has tried several antidepressants and is not completely satisfied with the results, additional medications may be tried in conjunction with an antidepressant. The drug lithium, which is commonly used to treat the psychiatric condition of bipolar disorder, may be prescribed with an antidepressant. Thyroid replacement medications are also sometimes added. Some believe that these medications may boost the effect of antidepressants although this is not well documented.

If a depressed patient is also markedly anxious, an anti-anxiety drug may be prescribed. Some psychiatrists will prescribe an anti-anxiety medication only at the beginning of treatment and then stop it when the person begins to improve on the antidepressant. Some psychiatrists may also briefly prescribe certain sleep medications then discontinue them once the depressed person begins to improve. A few psychiatrists may prescribe these medications for longer periods of time. There is concern about this practice, however, because of the possibility that the individual may grow overly reliant on this type of medication. For some people anti-anxiety drugs have the potential to become habit-forming. This is not the case, however, for antidepressants.

Electroconvulsive Therapy (ECT)

In some younger and older persons with serious depression, electroconvulsive therapy (ECT) may be used. ECT, sometimes referred to as shock therapy, does not have a very favorable image in the eyes of some. Movies that portray ECT as a dehumanizing punishment masquerading as treatment have created an unfavorable opinion about this procedure in the minds of the general public. The city of Berkeley, California, for example, banned the use of ECT a few years ago, although courts eventually overturned this local prohibition. Nevertheless, the idea of electric current being passed through the brain in order to help a person in emotional pain understandably creates a feeling of uneasiness in many people.

The fact is that ECT can be an extremely effective treatment. ECT is usually administered to individuals who have not responded to antidepressants or who cannot tolerate the side effects of those medications. It may also be used on an emergency basis for very severely depressed persons who have so neglected their health (for example, someone who has stopped eating) that they are in physical danger. It should never be administered to people with mild depressions or to those who are showing expectable reactions to life stresses.

A careful evaluation of the psychiatric, medical, and cognitive condition of the patient is made before administering ECT. When ECT is administered, the patient is rendered temporarily unconscious by the injection of an anesthetic. The patient is also administered other medications to paralyze muscles (which prevents sprains or bone fractures) and to control heart rate. Oxygen is given during the procedure. ECT involves the placement of two small electrodes on the skull through which an electrical current briefly passes for one or two seconds.

The preferred method (known as unilateral ECT) is to place both electrodes on the nondominant side of the skull. For right-handed persons this would typically be the right side. This method, in contrast to the placement of electrodes on opposite sides of the skull (bilateral ECT), is thought to reduce the frequency and severity of later memory complaints.

The effect of ECT is to induce a brain seizure that lasts 30 seconds to one minute. This procedure is repeated two to three times a week for a total of four to eight treatments. The number of treatments may vary depending on the patient's response. ECT has been shown to be effective in the vast majority of persons who receive it, and people usually improve more rapidly with ECT than with antidepressant medications.

A reasonable question does come to mind: Should such a procedure be administered to older people who may be in poor health or who have memory problems? The answer most experts give is a qualified yes, although people with cardiac disease must be carefully evaluated. ECT has been shown to be equally safe and effective for younger as well as older persons.

After ECT, patients are typically confused and disoriented for about an hour. During treatment and for a few weeks afterward, patients may show some memory difficulties. For the vast majority of persons, however, memory returns to normal. Despite the fact that researchers have not been able to conclusively demonstrate any negative long-term effects on memory, some individuals claim that they experience such problems. It is possible that for a small, select group of individuals, there are some mild, longer-term memory effects of ECT. Though there is some controversy about the impact of ECT on memory, it is important to note that most geriatric psychiatrists would not hesitate to use ECT with patients who are seriously depressed and for whom antidepressants were not useful.

The reason ECT helps depression is not well understood. It is presumed that brain seizure activity may change the balance of chemicals in the brain. Research is currently under way to try to better understand the reasons ECT is clinically useful.

INDIVIDUAL PSYCHOTHERAPY

Psychotherapy appears to be useful in alleviating clinical depression in younger and older people. In general, individual psychotherapy is the use of different psychological techniques by a mental health professional to change certain ways of feeling, thinking, or behaving that are experienced by the individual as unpleasant or undesirable. In principle, the therapist possesses the skills that can help the individual to achieve mutually agreed-upon goals. There are different schools of, or approaches to, psychotherapy, each of which has different theories about which aspects of experience are most critical to the formation and solving of various human problems. Although the usefulness of the most commonly recognized types of psychotherapy has been studied, no single approach has been found to be superior to the others. Some types of psychotherapy, however, have proven more effective than others in treating some problems among certain kinds of people.

Unfortunately, until recently, little research has evaluated the usefulness of psychotherapy for the elderly. This in part reflects the long-standing prejudice of some mental health professionals that psychotherapy would not be helpful to older people because, after a lifetime, it is believed unlikely they could or would want to change. This is, of course, a question that needs to be examined scientifically. What research is available, however, indicates that older people suffering from depression can benefit from psychotherapy.

Unfortunately, older people and their children may themselves share this therapeutic nihilism regarding the utility of psychotherapy for the aged. Older people often express the attitudes of the larger society that suggest that the aged are "too old to change." In addition, the current generation of older people has more negative attitudes about mental health care than younger persons do. For some older adults, receiving mental health services is seen as a source of shame and as something that will stigmatize them as "crazy." Others may believe that a visit to a mental health professional is the first step toward institutionalization. As discussed earlier, an older adult's initial confusion or apprehension about psychotherapy may be the first critical issue that must be addressed in treatment. If the older adult is unclear about the purpose of psychotherapy it is unlikely that he or she will participate in it. The same may be true for spouses or adult children, who usually play an important role in bringing the patient for treatment. The family must be educated about the nature and goals of psychotherapy.

Some researchers have found among younger persons that the most effective treatment for depression is a combination of antidepressants and psychotherapy. For older people suffering from major depression, it is important that consideration be given to the use of antidepressant medication even if they are already receiving psychotherapy.

On the other hand, some older adults are only treated with antidepressant medication when they very much need psychotherapy. Although antidepressant medications may be very effective in initially alleviating the most serious symptoms of depression, the causes of the condition may remain unchanged. Patients may be at risk for the recurrence of a major depression if they have not dealt with life circumstances that precipitated the depression in the first place.

There are several different approaches to psychotherapy. Only the most common methods will be discussed here.

Supportive Psychotherapy

Supportive psychotherapy does not derive from a particular theoretical point of view. It reflects more general efforts by the therapist to provide support, encouragement, and acceptance to the older person. Individuals may have few persons to whom they can turn for support and validation. Some older people report a significant change in mood after only brief supportive counseling.

Working with a therapist, the older person may be better able to clarify the scope and extent of current problems as well as his or her own social and personal assets. The individual may learn to look at things somewhat differently, to try out some new possibilities, and to make better sense of life. Although some may regard the psychotherapy relationship as similar to friendship, it is in many ways different. The therapist does not have personal and social expectations about what the older person should do for him or her. One of the problems faced by some older adults is that they feel family members or friends do not want to listen to them. Or they may find that the response to what they say is not helpful. Such situations can lead to feelings of isolation, loss of perspective on perceived problems, a sense of helplessness, and depressive feelings.

> Fay Johnson, a well-dressed and carefully coifed 65-year-old widow, began her first therapy session by cataloguing her social and cultural activities. She claimed to be managing her senior years "marvelously" and felt "sorry" about all those "truly old people who lead such dreadful lives." When asked why she had sought treatment at a geriatric mental health clinic she vaguely referred to some "family problems" that needed to be "cleared up."
>
> By her third psychotherapy session she reluctantly admitted that things were not so marvelous and that she had been intermittently depressed for two years. Her

emotional difficulties began when she learned that her
daughter was drug-addicted and living a marginal
lifestyle. She felt that she could tell no one about this
because of the deep embarrassment it caused her.

After three months of weekly meetings Mrs. Johnson
reported feeling "relieved," less depressed, and less
focused on her daughter. During the supportive sessions
she better clarified feelings toward her daughter, the
extent to which she could or could not help her
daughter, and whom she might trust with her "secret."

For older adults with incapacitating major depressions, supportive psychotherapy may provide a kind of support that may not be available elsewhere. Researchers have found that depression may damage close relationships and that as depression continues people may distance themselves from the depressed individual. Since the therapist is not personally involved with the depressed person, he or she may be better able to tolerate the kinds of behavior that others find aversive. The therapist may also play a key role in helping the depressed person to continue to take antidepressant medications that may have been prescribed. In view of the side effects that frequently accompany these medications, some older people need active encouragement to continue to take them. Emotional support from the therapist may make the critical difference.

Mental health professionals sometimes find that older people with, for example, ongoing personality problems, difficult life circumstances, or health problems that are accompanied by chronic depression may benefit by a long-term supportive relationship that helps them to maintain their emotional equilibrium and consequently prevents more serious depressive episodes. Other mental health professionals report that as the older person begins to feel better emotionally and develops trust in the therapist and more confidence in his or her own ability to tackle existing problems, supportive therapy can be the foundation for the development of a more focused psychological intervention. Although the frequency and variety of techniques used by geriatric therapists have not been been carefully studied, many therapists probably use variants of supportive therapy. Since supportive therapy does not have an explicit theoretical focus, little research has systematically examined its impact on the emotional and functional abilities of older individuals. Much more work needs to be done.

Psychodynamic Psychotherapy

As discussed earlier, psychodynamically oriented mental health professionals often view depression not so much as the problem but as the symptom of underlying conflicts or problems about which the individual may not be aware. One form of therapeutic work with a psychodynamic focus is psychoanalysis. Psychoanalysis is an attempt to explore early life experiences and their present effects on a person. It is usually a costly intensive and extensive treatment (three sessions a week for several years is typical). Few persons and even fewer older people actually use this form of treatment. There are briefer forms of treatment that have psychodynamic underpinnings. Most persons treated by psychodynamically oriented therapists will be seen once or twice a week for a period of a few months or sometimes years. There are even briefer forms of this type of psychotherapy that have a definite time limit—for example, six sessions.

Psychoanalysis and psychodynamic therapy have not been well researched. In large measure this lack of research is because it is difficult to verify the early childhood experiences of an adult and to measure the complex processes that psychodynamic theory suggest go on within the mind. Although a sizable number of mental health professionals who do psychotherapy with older people have been influenced by psychodynamic theory, only a few studies have specifically examined its usefulness for older adults. Some mental health professionals working with the aged report that older people have greatly profited by this form of therapy.

> Claire Ackerman, an extremely articulate and intelligent 82-year-old woman, complained of feelings of depression that still persisted two years after her husband had died. She was puzzled why "this bereavement thing" had not yet ended. "After all," she said dispassionately, "I must get on with life." After several months of psychodynamically oriented therapy, it became apparent that Mrs. Ackerman had felt depressed on and off throughout

her life. Despite her intelligence and many accomplish-
ments, she felt deeply insecure about her intellectual and
interpersonal capabilities. She had had a conflict-ridden
relationship with her husband that was better
characterized by anger than affection.

As she became more comfortable with and capable of
discussing distressing feelings, she turned to early
experiences — "things I haven't thought about in years."
When discussing how difficult it was for her to fully
experience feelings, she recalled the demands of caring
for her ailing mother when she was only a child. "Don't
ever get angry at your mother or make too much noise,"
she recalled her father admonishing her. "It might kill
her." While exploring ongoing feelings of being socially
awkward, she remembered the sense of social isolation
that had resulted from being one of the few Jewish
people in a predominantly Italian neighborhood.

These and other insights from childhood were an
impetus to change her present behavior with others. In
the course of a year and a half of psychotherapy she
overcame her depression, expanded the scope and quality
of her relationships with friends, and mended a difficult
relationship with her two daughters. Mrs. Ackerman
spoke of the growing emotional satisfaction she derived
from interacting with others. "Who would have thought
that a person my age could change so much," she
remarked toward the end of psychotherapy. "I wish I
would have done this earlier in my life."

One specialized approach to psychotherapy with the aged, discussed by Dr. Robert Butler, is reminiscence therapy. Dr. Butler
argues that some persons, with increasing awareness of the relative shortness of life, will engage in a process of life review that
is emotionally beneficial. The individual may examine issues,
conflicts, concerns, and triumphs from earlier phases of life.

Behavioral and Cognitive Therapies

Perhaps the best researched and most carefully developed psychotherapy for depressed elderly people has been completed by
psychologists Larry Thompson and Dolores Gallagher. They

have used techniques developed for younger persons and adapted them to the special needs and concerns of older people. In general, their research has demonstrated that supportive, psychodynamic, cognitive, and behavioral therapies all show promise in alleviating depression problems in older people. Cognitive and behavioral therapies, however, appear to be especially effective in helping older people stay free from depression.

As noted earlier, behaviorally oriented psychologists believe that people's emotional well-being is tied to their behavior and the consequences of their behavior. An older person who has stopped engaging in previously pleasurable activities or interactions may become depressed. Drs. Thompson and Gallagher have developed a structured behavioral therapy program for depressed older people designed to increase pleasurable activities and interactions and decrease aversive ones. In contrast to psychodynamic therapy—which may involve a wide-ranging exploration of past and present thoughts, feelings, and behaviors—behavior therapy often follows a fairly well defined series of steps.

At first the older person is educated about the role of behavior in affecting emotions. The frequency of positive and negative events in the older person's immediate environment is evaluated. The patient is also asked to monitor his or her mood on a day-to-day basis and examine the effect of behaviors on mood. The older person is then encouraged to increase or decrease certain activities based on their emotional impact. After the behavior therapy sessions are completed, progress is reviewed and assistance is offered to help the older person to continue to apply what has been learned. Sometimes "booster sessions" are scheduled later to solve any difficulties that may have come up.

Drs. Thompson and Gallagher have also modified a cognitive therapy program for older adults developed by psychiatrist Aaron Beck and his associates. As in behavioral therapy, older people are educated about the principles that will be applied in the treatment. In this case, people are taught about the relationship between certain patterns of thinking and the way people feel. Older adults are taught to identify their own patterns of negative thinking and are then asked to monitor these patterns and their own moods on a daily basis. Once this is done, older people are shown how certain kinds of negative thinking are actually distortions of the truth. Patients are asked to try other ways of thinking about experiences. These new ways of thinking should help to reduce depression. Like behavior therapy, cognitive therapy is also time-limited. Some persons may continue for longer periods of time and begin to examine lifelong beliefs that probably have negative effects on mood (such as, "I've never really accomplished anything worthwhile in my life"). It is important to note that some therapists use cognitive and behavioral approaches in conjunction.

While on the whole these techniques appear useful for older people, some older individuals may not benefit. Or an older person might benefit from one technique but not another. The goal of research is to determine what kind of therapy is most effective for persons confronted by various problems.

James Larson came to the geriatric mental health clinic complaining of having felt very depressed for two years. He was diagnosed with a major depression. He had been treated by a private psychiatrist for one year with antidepressant medication, but, after reviewing his treatment, the clinic psychiatrist concluded that Mr. Larson had never received an adequate dosage of medication.

After two months of more appropriate antidepressant treatment than he had previously received, Mr. Larson reported feeling better but continued to feel mild to moderately depressed and to evidence a pattern of negative thinking that appeared to be linked with the depressive feelings. For example, despite the fact that Mr. Larson was quite accomplished at virtually all aspects of home repair and maintenance, he focused only on his failures. Once, after attempting a major plumbing repair, he realized he needed the assistance of a professional. He saw this as evidence of his "stupidity" and declining talents.

Using cognitive therapy techniques, the therapist asked Mr. Larson to monitor his thoughts and feelings. A clear pattern of negative thinking and depressed mood emerged. Although skeptical at first, the documented relationship between his thoughts and his moods encouraged Mr. Larson to further examine his thinking patterns. The propensity to label any difficulties in home repair projects as evidence of his "stupidity" was examined. He gradually conceded that, indeed, he did have certain abilities and that perhaps he was being "too hard on myself." Gradually Mr. Larson showed an increasing ability to monitor and control negative thoughts—with concurrent improvement in his mood.

Group, Couple, and Family Psychotherapies

The general principles of individual psychotherapy have been adapted to different formats. Psychotherapy can be done in groups, with couples, and with whole families. Each of these different approaches is thought to have specific therapeutic advantages.

Psychologists have documented over the years that groups of persons have the potential to influence people's feelings, attitudes, and behaviors. Group psychotherapy uses peer influence for the purpose of psychological change. Many groups are organized for persons experiencing the same kind of problem—for example, depression. An individual participating in such a group may get information, receive direct feedback on how his or her behavior affects others, learn better ways to cope with problems, have an opportunity to express feelings, experience a new sense of hope, and gain a sense of belonging. Drs. Gallagher and Thompson (mentioned earlier) use the group format to conduct "classes" with a cognitive and behavioral focus that teach older people how to better cope with depression.

In couple psychotherapy two individuals meet with a therapist to focus on common problems. With older people these meetings are usually used for a marriage partner or for an aging parent and an adult child. Older married couples may complain that their relationship is unsatisfying and want to change or improve it. Sometimes difficulties have existed for many years, or they may be more recent. Retirement or physical or mental illness in one of the partners may precipitate strains in the relationship. If one of the partners is depressed, marital strains may make it more difficult for the depressed person to adequately recover from depression.

Carl Hendriks and his wife, Sonia, admitted that their relationship had never been particularly satisfying for either of them. There had been ongoing disagreement about how to raise the children, unhappiness with their sexual relationship, and a general feeling that they were "mismatched." Mr. Hendriks had been diagnosed with a variety of medical problems in the last few years that limited his mobility. In addition, he had been feeling depressed for the last year but was advised that, because of his medical condition, antidepressants would not be prescribed. Mr. Hendriks's physical and emotional difficulties had clearly put a further strain on an already problematic relationship. During a recent argument, for example, Mr. Hendriks had struck his wife. He was shocked and ashamed by his behavior. Both Mr. and Mrs. Hendriks agreed that it was time to seek marital counseling.

They both felt that if they were younger they would probably have divorced, but given their advanced years, they did not want to do this. Their goal was to "learn how to live with each other."

The therapist used a modified behavioral therapy approach to improve their relationship. He helped both Mr. and Mrs. Hendriks to identify behaviors on the other's part that were upsetting or provocative and those behaviors that were pleasing or satisfying. Each was asked to make efforts to reduce unpleasant and increase pleasant behaviors. For example, since the Hendrikses both enjoyed cultural activities, they were asked to increase the frequency with which they attended such events.

Over time, the frequency of arguments decreased while the number of satisfying interactions increased between them. The Hendrikses reported a positive improvement in the "atmosphere" of their relationship and, for the first time in many years, experienced feelings of affection for each other. Concurrently, Mr. Hendriks said that he felt much less depressed despite continuing physical health problems.

Older people and their adult children may similarly seek to improve long-standing relationship problems—or wish to deal with difficulties that have recently emerged. As will be discussed later, adult children of older people with mood disorders may be especially interested in psychotherapeutic meetings to address difficulties often prompted by these emotional problems.

Another vehicle for trying to better deal with problems is family psychotherapy. This method has become increasingly popular in the last 20 years. Although there are a variety of approaches to family psychotherapy, many mental health professionals believe that families are characterized by complex systems of interrelationships that may inadvertently create or sustain problems in one or more of their members. Often a family will enter therapy because one member has problems that concern all of them. Family therapists may see the manifest problem of one family member as part of a larger pattern of difficulties that, in one way or another, affect all family members. By addressing such underlying family difficulties the well-being of the family as a whole will improve.

THE SETTING FOR TREATMENT

Treatment for clinical depression may take place on an outpatient or inpatient basis. Outpatient treatment may be in a clinic or in the private office of a health professional. A variety of factors may determine the choice of setting.

Most people are treated for depression as outpatients—that is, they continue living in the community and make regular visits to the office of a mental health professional for treatment. Probably a large number of older people receive treatment for depression from the physician who sees them for medical problems. Since older people usually discuss a variety of concerns with their doctors, a nonpsychiatric physician is often the first health professional to whom symptoms of depression will be presented. In practice, studies have shown that nonpsychiatric physicians often fail to diagnose clinical depression in older people when it exists. Some physicians, of course, competently diagnose and treat mental health problems in the elderly. Some have argued that if a mental health professional is available, the older person should be referred to him or her or, at the least, should receive treatment from a mental health professional in conjunction with treatment from the physician.

A good private mental health professional will evaluate the medical, social, and psychological factors discussed earlier that are relevant to depression. If the professional is inexperienced or is incapable of making this evaluation, referral for consultation with a geriatric specialist should be made. For example, a psychologist treating an older person for major depression would want to make sure that the older adult has had a recent medical examination and has been evaluated to determine if antidepressant medications should be prescribed.

Services may also be provided in an outpatient mental health clinic or community mental health center. The advantage of this arrangement is that such clinics typically have a variety of mental health professionals available in one place or have other professionals to whom they frequently make referrals for consultations. There are a few specialized geriatric mental health clinics that provide comprehensive services to older people and their families. Usually clinic care is less expensive than private care.

Sometimes, however, treatment for depression will take place in an inpatient setting. There are a variety of inpatient settings. For example, a general hospital may have a special unit devoted to the treatment of psychiatric problems; some medical centers have large psychiatric divisions; some psychiatric hospitals are "free-standing"—that is, they are not part of a medical center but may use the services of a nearby medical center; and some medical centers or psychiatric hospitals have specialized geriatric units with personnel knowledgeable about issues in treating older people with psychiatric problems. The length of time an individual is hospitalized depends on a number of factors, but in recent years the amount of time has been decreasing. An average length of stay is three to six weeks. In an inpatient setting the older person typically receives a variety of psychiatric, psychological, social work, and recreational rehabilitation services. On discharge from the inpatient service, the older patient should be referred for continuing care on an outpatient basis. Some institutions have outpatient clinics that work in coordination with the inpatient service.

The choice of treatment setting depends on a number of factors. People will usually be hospitalized if there is any significant concern that they may attempt suicide. Some older people's clinical depressions may not have responded well to outpatient treatment. They will therefore be hospitalized to be treated with new medication in a setting where their progress and any drug side effects may be closely monitored. For example, depressed older adults with medical problems (most notably cardiac difficulties) might be hospitalized if antidepressants are prescribed because of the need to evaluate any adverse effects of these medications. Some older people are so emotionally and socially debilitated by depression that it is useful to temporarily place them in a structured setting with many supports. Similarly, most persons who are judged in need of ECT are hospitalized.

Effectiveness of Treatments

A critical question is: How effective are different treatments for depression in older adults? Unfortunately, a clear answer to this question is hampered by the lack of research. The definitions of clinical depression and the treatments that are available have changed over the years. In addition, the quality of studies varies considerably. Effectiveness of treatment has been defined by studies in many different ways. Should one, for example, consider a treatment successful if an older person with a major depression significantly improved but then had another episode of depression one year later?

In general, evaluation of the effectiveness of treatment has been approached by determining the degree to which a depressed older person was treated and: (1) got better and stayed better, (2) got better but then became depressed again, or (3) never really got better. But the answer to these questions also depends on the setting in which the older person received treatment. People who are psychiatrically hospitalized tend to have more serious cases of depression than those who are treated on an outpatient basis. It is possible that hospitalized patients may not respond as well to treatment as do outpatients.

Among older people treated for depression on an inpatient basis, only about one-third get better and stay better. Most of the remaining individuals get better but have additional episodes of depression. A small portion of patients (estimates vary) never fully recover from clinical depression. Among older adults treated on an outpatient basis, one-third to one-half get better and stay better. As with elderly treated on an inpatient basis, most of the rest get better but have additional episodes of depression, and a small number never fully recover.

It is difficult to determine which mental health treatment is most effective in helping older adults with depression since often pharmacotherapy and psychotherapy (and sometimes ECT) are given together. Among older persons treated in an inpatient setting there are usually a variety of psychological, social, and somatic (antidepressants and/or ECT) treatments simultaneously provided. It is reasonable to assume that pharmacotherapy, ECT, and psychotherapy each make a contribution to improving depression in older people—and that a combination of treatments might be most useful. Among outpatient depressed older adults, both antidepressant medication and cognitive-behavioral therapy have been proven useful in alleviating depression.

It is important to note that even though a fairly large proportion of older adults treated for depression have additional episodes, treatment can significantly shorten the duration of the episodes and, in the case of ongoing treatment, can probably reduce the number of episodes from what would have been experienced if there had been no treatment. Unfortunately, clinical depression may be a chronic illness that needs to be managed for life. Without treatment, life for the patient and his or her family would be much more difficult.

Bipolar Disorder and Cyclothymia

Definition

A tragic irony is that some persons who experience periods of serious depression also have episodes of mania, in which they may feel especially good, cheerful, happy, "high," or, sometimes, irritable. The feeling of being manic is quite different from the usual enthusiasm or excitement that people feel when life circumstances are favorable. During manic episodes the individual's judgment may be seriously impaired and his or her behavior may have negative repercussions for his or her life. An individual who has experienced one or more episodes of mania is diagnosed with bipolar disorder. Bipolar disorder (*bipolar* indicates the two different emotional poles) was formerly called manic depression. The vast majority of persons who have had manic episodes have also had depressive episodes. Occasionally, however, persons with bipolar disorder report having only had episodes of mania. Manic episodes occur over various lengths of time. In part, the length of a manic episode depends on how soon the individual receives treatment. The episode will eventually end on its own, however, and sometimes is followed by depression. The psychiatric diagnostic manual, *DSM-III-R,* generally defines an episode of mania in the following way.

1. There is a clearly defined period of elevated or irritable mood; the individual may experience this as being "on top of the world," "cheerful," "high," or something similar. Less frequently, there are feelings of irritability or hostility.

2. During this period of changed mood, the individual must report at least three of the symptoms described below (four if the individual's predominant mood is that of irritability):

   Inflated self-esteem: This is an exaggerated sense of oneself or one's abilities that may seriously distort reality.

   Reduced need for sleep: The individual may feel refreshed even after only a few hours of sleep.

   Unusually talkative or a feeling of "pressure" to keep talking.

   Rapid shifting of ideas or the experience that thoughts are racing.

   Easy distractibility.

   Increased activity.

   Involvement in activities that have the potential for serious consequences. This may include spending large sums of money, increasing sexual activity, or putting oneself in dangerous circumstances.

3. There is damage or impairment in ability to work, engage in social activities, and/or carry on relationships with others, or the need to be hospitalized.

4. There have not been delusions or hallucinations that existed without the presence of changed mood.

5. The current condition does not coexist with other disorders that are primarily characterized by symptoms of a psychosis such as schizophrenia.

6. The present condition is not caused by an organic factor, for example, an underlying medical problem.

Manic episodes are further characterized by their severity and, if accompanied by psychotic features, by the nature of these features. Of particular interest is the presence of delusions. A less severe form of a manic episode is called hypomania. Mania and hypomania are similar except that in hypomania symptoms tend to be less severe, delusions are not present, and the episode does not clearly cause problems in functioning on the job, in social activities, or with others.

Cyclothymia is another type of mood disorder that is less severe than bipolar disorder. It is an ongoing disturbance of mood in which the individual has periods of hypomania and periods when there are symptoms of depression. To be diagnosed with cyclothymia, *DSM-III-R* specifies that:

1. For adults, there must be a minimum of two years in which there have been many periods of hypomania and periods of depressed mood, decreased interest in things, or lessened pleasure (but not so severe as to meet the criteria for major depression).

2. For the previous two years, while experiencing the above mood changes, the individual has not been without hypomanic or depressive symptoms for a period longer than two months.

3. The individual did not experience a major depression or manic episode within the first two years of the disturbance in mood.

4. A psychiatric disorder like schizophrenia is not present.

5. The above problems cannot be the result of an organic factor.

There is very little research on bipolar disorder in older people and virtually none on cyclothymia in the elderly. Bipolar disorder in older adults appears, however, to be similar to that seen in younger persons. Some mental health professionals have noted that, when manic, older people may look more confused, cognitively impaired, paranoid, and agitated than younger persons. Their moods may also tend to be more irritable or show a greater mixture of depressed mood and manic mood than those of younger people. The vast majority of older people with bipolar disorder have had it for many years. Most bipolar disorder— that is, the first appearance of mania—is diagnosed between the ages of 20 and 40. Cases of a first manic episode in late life have been reported but they are not common. The appearance of manic symptoms in late life, however, may signal underlying medical problems. Some geriatric mental health professionals report that older people with lifelong histories of bipolar disorder tend to have more severe and more frequent episodes of mania as they get older. More research is needed, however, to document the course of both bipolar disorder and cyclothymia over the life span.

Frequency and Possible Causes

Bipolar disorder afflicts about 1–2 percent of the population (with a similar prevalence in older and younger adults). Older people with bipolar disorder represent only a relatively small percentage of patients seen by inpatient and outpatient mental health professionals. Most mental health professionals believe bipolar disorder has a strong genetic component. Studies have shown that close relatives of a person with bipolar disorder are much more likely to also have the illness. How this genetic variation predisposes the brain to poorly regulate mood is not well understood; research continues to be done. Though the condition is genetic in origin, certain life stresses may well trigger an episode of mania.

Evaluation

As with an evaluation for any mental disorder, a past and current history of the problem must be taken; medical tests must be requested; and an understanding of the person's social, psychological, and family circumstances should be obtained. In addition to the kinds of tests required for depression, a neurological examination; an electroencephalogram (EEG), which measures certain aspects of brain activity; and tests for proper kidney functioning are often recommended. Since the medication most frequently prescribed for bipolar disorder, lithium, may have effects on the thyroid gland and kidneys, a baseline (before treatment) measure of their functioning can be useful.

Treatment

SOMATIC TREATMENTS

In the 1950s it was found that the drug lithium significantly helped people with bipolar disorder. In fact, for many people who had suffered the nightmarish ups and downs of this illness, lithium was regarded as a miracle drug. Research has indeed shown that lithium plays a significant role in controlling mania and depression in the majority of people with bipolar disorder. However, as they must when prescribing antidepressants, psychiatrists must take special precautions in prescribing lithium because of some of the biological changes associated with aging. For example, lithium is stored in the body's water, so higher concentrations of it tend to develop in older people because they have a smaller proportion of water (relative to body size) than do younger persons. Older people may also eliminate lithium from their systems less efficiently because kidney function becomes less efficient with advancing age.

The amount of lithium that is in a person's system is measured by its concentration in the blood. Since persons taking lithium may run the danger of getting too much of the drug, they should be required to take regular blood tests. Older people are prescribed less lithium than younger persons. The amount of lithium an individual may need may also fluctuate. For example, during the summer, when people are more likely to perspire, they may need less lithium.

There are a variety of possible side effects of lithium that should be monitored closely. Confusion—and other cognitive symptoms—are side effects that should be very closely watched in the aged. Occasionally a mental health professional may mistakenly regard these symptoms as part of the aging process or as evidence of dementia. If these symptoms appear, a psychiatrist will usually decrease or discontinue the medication for a week or two. Lithium may also be associated with certain cardiac irregularities, may cause increased urination, and, in some persons, may cause kidney problems. People who take lithium for long periods of time may develop a condition called hypothyroidism (inadequate thyroid functioning). With care, these difficulties can be managed.

Some people taking lithium also complain of upset stomach, diarrhea, and similar problems. These side effects are sometimes alleviated by reducing medication or prescribing other types of lithium. Psoriasis (a skin disruption) has also been associated with lithium use.

Since most persons with bipolar disorder will be required to take lithium throughout their lives, managing the side effects of the medication is an important role for the psychiatrist. If problems with side effects are not effectively dealt with, the patient may stop taking lithium. This puts him or her at greater risk for an episode of mania or depression. Given the variety of medical problems that typically accompany aging, management of side effects—and monitoring of potential interactions of lithium with other medications—requires vigilance by the psychiatrist.

Maria Silva, an elderly woman with a lifelong history of bipolar disorder, was engaged in a lively conversation with other patients in the clinic waiting room. "Hello, my friend the doctor!" she exclaimed as her psychiatrist, with whom she had an appointment, approached her. As Mrs. Silva walked to the psychiatrist's office, she told an off-color joke and then poked the psychiatrist when he did not laugh as heartily as she did.

"Things are just fine," said Mrs. Silva enthusiastically. She detailed her many activities of the last two weeks.

She had been considerably more active than usual. She discussed "new thoughts" she had about her life and concluded, "If there were more people like me, the world would be a better place. I've been thinking about calling the president to give him some new ideas on how to achieve world peace."

After considerable probing by the psychiatrist, Mrs. Silva admitted that she had stopped taking lithium because of an exacerbation of psoriasis and weight gain. "After all," said Mrs. Silva confidently, "I should know what's best for me!" Mrs. Silva agreed to restart lithium, however, and within two weeks her manic symptoms subsided.

If a person is in a manic episode, it is sometimes necessary to treat him or her with a class of drugs call neuroleptics. These are also called major tranquilizers and have been proven useful in cutting short manic episodes. Most psychiatrists will try to use these drugs briefly since they have been associated with a condition called tardive dyskinesia (TD). TD is a usually permanent side effect of neuroleptics that is found in a fairly large number of people who are treated with these medications on an ongoing basis—these are usually people with schizophrenia. Recent research suggests that older people may be particularly susceptible to developing TD. Despite this, some people with bipolar disorder must be treated on an ongoing basis with neuroleptics if they do not respond adequately to lithium.

As noted earlier, electroconvulsive therapy (ECT) is sometimes used to treat serious depression. It can also be used to treat manic episodes. Typically ECT will be used when the person has not adequately responded to lithium, neuroleptics, or a combination of these medications. Occasionally ECT is given immediately, in cases of very severe manic episodes when it is critical that symptoms diminish rapidly.

The drug carbamazepine (trade name Tegretol) has been used separately and in combination with lithium. An anticonvulsant, carbamazepine is sometimes prescribed when the individual has not responded adequately to lithium and/or neuroleptics. Further research is needed to better determine the usefulness of carbamazepine for bipolar disorder.

PSYCHOTHERAPY

An older person suffering from bipolar disorder may profit from
some form of psychotherapy. Although the preponderance of
scientific evidence indicates that bipolar disorder is a biologically
based disturbance in mood, the manner in which an individual
copes with daily stresses may reduce the likelihood of future psychiatric episodes. Supportive therapy may be especially useful in
problem-solving the sometimes complex social and personal consequences that follow episodes of psychiatric illness. It may also
help the patient to learn how to appropriately view other social
relationships, to try different ways of dealing with the need to take
psychiatric medications for many years, and to more generally
come to terms with this difficult illness. For older adults, couple or
family psychotherapy may be helpful in mending relationships
damaged by episodes of mania and depression, educating family
members about bipolar disorder, and teaching both patient and
family how future episodes may be more profitably managed.

THE SETTING FOR TREATMENT

Whether the depression or mania of bipolar disorder should be
treated on an inpatient or outpatient basis is generally dictated
by the same guidelines outlined earlier for major depression. In
a manic episode, an individual may be particularly at risk
because personal judgment may be seriously impaired and the
individual may be involved in activities that pose harm to him- or
herself. In this case, the patient may be hospitalized. This is
typically done with the patient's consent. Sometimes, however, if
the patient is judged a significant risk to himself or others, in
most states he may be temporarily yet involuntarily committed.
States have varying legal procedures surrounding involuntary
commitment. Most psychiatrists much prefer that the person
voluntarily enter the hospital, and family members may be effectively utilized to encourage the patient to do so.

Effectiveness of Treatments

Few studies have examined the effectiveness of different treatments for bipolar disorder in older adults. The main focus of
treatment in younger persons has been lithium. It is possible that

lithium may be as effective for older adults as it is for younger persons (70–80 percent of younger people show a positive response to lithium).

Mood Disorders and the Family

Depression and bipolar disorder, like most psychiatric difficulties, can place enormous strain on existing relationships. Several years ago psychologist Myrna Weissman and her colleagues studied the impacts on the relationships of women who were diagnosed with depression. They found that depression damaged close relationships. Even after the women recovered from depression they continued to have interpersonal problems, especially with their spouses. Recent research by this author has documented that spouses and adult children caring for older adults with major depression show high levels of emotional stress and are often unsure about how to help the afflicted older person. Not only are some family members deeply troubled by witnessing this emotional distress in someone they love, but also they may grow frustrated when their continuing efforts to help seem to make little difference. When depressed, an individual may ask for comfort, reassurance, and support, yet reject well-intentioned efforts by the family member to help. Over the course of a lengthy illness, the family member may lose patience and even grow angry with the older adult and, subsequently, feel guilty about having such feelings.

The way the family responds to the depressed person, however, may make a difference in how quickly the patient recovers. Researchers have found that certain ways of interacting with depressed individuals make a difference in the patient's recovery. In recent years several new approaches to working with the families of depressed persons have been reported. One of these, interpersonal psychotherapy, was developed by psychologist Myrna Weissman and psychiatrist Gerald Klerman, in part because of Dr. Weissman's research on the negative effects of depression on close relationships. Other existing psychotherapeutic approaches, including cognitive, behavioral, and marital therapies, have been adapted to deal with the interpersonal difficulties associated with depression. This is a promising area of current research and clinical practice.

Chapter 2

Cognitive Problems

Organic Mental Syndromes

- A syndrome is a group of characteristic problems the cause of which is not necessarily known.

- Two organic mental syndromes most often seen in older adults are dementia and delirium.

- Dementia refers to deficits in short-term and long-term memory often accompanied by difficulties in thinking and judgment, personality changes, and other cognitive problems.

- Delirium involves problems with maintaining and shifting attention, with logical thinking, and with speech as well as other difficulties.

- An individual may have delirium as well as dementia.

- Until recently most studies have suggested that 4% of persons 65 years or older have "severe" dementia; very recent research suggests that this figure may be even higher.

- Evaluation of delirium and dementia includes a careful investigation of the individual's cognitive problems, medical status, and life circumstances.

Organic Mental Disorders

- An organic mental disorder is a specific mental syndrome the cause of which is known or can be assumed to be known.

- Two of the most common types of organic mental disorders in which a dementia syndrome is present are primary degenerative dementia of the Alzheimer type (Alzheimer's disease) and multi-infarct dementia.

- The cause of Alzheimer's disease is not known, although there are genetic, viral, environmental, and immunological theories regarding the subject. Many of these theories have been or are currently being researched.

- The cause of multi-infarct dementia is a series of small strokes that over time damage brain tissue.

- There are many possible causes of delirium including certain medical problems and some medications or combinations of medications.

- Treatment for delirium involves finding and treating its underlying cause(s).

- Although most dementias are irreversible, certain medications and some forms of psychological treatment may be used to manage the problems associated with the condition.

- Research is currently examining whether some drugs might improve the mental abilities of people with dementia. So far, however, none has been shown to significantly improve mental abilities.

- Family members caring for people with dementia play a critical caretaking role yet face considerable practical and emotional stresses.

Introduction

Perhaps the most profound ability of the human mind is the capacity to experience a distinctive sense of self. A critical component of the sense of self is memory, because the self is built on the expanding history of personal experiences that are catalogued in memory. Without memory the individual inhabits a world of unconnected moments, resulting in a tenuous sense of self defined only by the ever-changing pushes and pulls of the environment. The progressive loss of mental abilities that occurs in some older adults—most notably, the loss of memory—is one of life's cruelest tragedies because it robs the individual of one of evolution's greatest gifts—the sense of self.

Mental decline has been called many names: senile dementia, senility, hardening of the arteries, Alzheimer's disease, and organic brain syndrome. Although these terms are frequently used imprecisely, they all refer to the loss of cognitive capacity that occurs in later life. Despite the deep suffering that cognitive loss causes both for people with this problem and for their families, the topic was virtually ignored by professionals until recently. The reasons for this are many, but in part it reflects a more general discounting of problems of older people, ignorance of brain functioning, and the false belief that mental decline was an inevitable part of growing older. In the last few years, however, in part because of the increasing proportion of elderly people in the U.S. population, the problem of dementia has received considerable attention in the public media and has been the focus of growing concern by researchers and health care providers. While this attention is a welcome sign, it has unfortunately generated unfounded fears among some older people that they are at great risk for significant loss of mental capacity. The fact is that only a small percentage of older adults have conditions like Alzheimer's disease. For those who have this condition and their families, however, it is one of the biggest challenges they will ever face.

In this chapter different losses of mental or cognitive abilities in late life will be discussed. Questions frequently asked about this topic by older individuals and their families will be addressed, including:

What is cognitive loss? Are there different kinds of it?

How common is the condition? Are close relatives of people with cognitive loss more likely to suffer from it in the later years than others are?

What is the cause of cognitive loss?

How do mental health professionals diagnose cognitive loss?

Can anything be done to improve or even cure cognitive loss?

How do families cope with caring for a relative with cognitive loss?

What happens to people with cognitive loss over the long run?

Normal Aging of the Human Brain

The different brain capacities necessary for daily functioning have mostly been studied by neuropsychologists and neurologists—professionals who specialize in the evaluation and measurement of brain function. Some of the primary mental abilities in which neuropsychologists and neurologists are usually interested include concentration, short-term and long-term memory, visual-spatial capacity, and abstract reasoning. Concentration is the ability to actively attend to things such as listening to a conversation or reading a book. Learning new information, for example, becomes very difficult if an individual cannot concentrate. Short-term memory is the capacity to retain newly learned information for brief periods of time. One example is the ability to recall facts that were conveyed a few minutes earlier. Long-term memory is the ability to recall information acquired in the past, for example, things that happened several days or even several years ago. Visual-spatial ability encompasses the capacity to orient oneself in the environment. Finding one's way to a familiar destination in part requires visual-spatial ability. Abstract reasoning is mirrored by a wide range of mental activities that includes the abilities to integrate, compare, and synthesize ideas or concepts. For example, the ability to recognize that a rolling pin and a frying pan share the common characteristic of being kitchen utensils is a basic part of abstract reasoning.

Measures such as intelligence tests (IQ tests) are an attempt to generally quantify some of the above and other mental abilities. For many years it was assumed that mental abilities naturally declined with age. Researchers found, for example, that older people scored lower on IQ tests than younger individuals. Researchers later recognized, however, that these lower IQ scores generally reflected the more limited educational opportunities that had been available to people of the older generation and did not necessarily indicate age-related declines in intelligence. Researchers also found that poor performance in some tests of mental ability simply reflected the fact that older people worked more slowly at completing the tests; if the older people were given additional time, their performance was comparable to that of younger persons. Although scientists have concluded that certain mental abilities do indeed decline with age, especially when people become very old, on the whole these changes do not significantly affect older people's day-to-day lives. It is noteworthy that there are considerable individual differences in these changes and that the mental abilities of some persons actually increase as they age.

Abnormal Changes in the Brain

The fact that some persons evidence considerable impairment of mental functions in later life has been recorded since the time of the early Greeks. Until very recently, such impairment was assumed to be part of a general process of brain degeneration caused by aging. This assumption was challenged by researchers in England in the late 1960s. B. E. Tomlinson and colleagues evaluated the mental abilities of a group of middle-aged and older persons over several years. Some individuals evidenced clinically significant cognitive loss. When people in the study died, the researchers did brain autopsies to determine whether there were differences between the brains of persons with cognitive loss and those of persons without cognitive loss. What they found was contrary to the then popular belief that most cognitive loss in late life was caused by hardening of the arteries, which was believed to restrict blood flow to the brain. Their studies revealed that the most common characteristics of people who had dementia were brain changes that were the same as those described by German neurologist Alois Alzheimer in the early twentieth century (later called Alzheimer's disease). Alzheimer's disease was thought at that time, however, to afflict only younger individuals. Dr. Tomlinson and his research group forced the medical world to begin to re-examine some basic assumptions about mental functioning and aging that, in retrospect, had little scientific data to support them.

The pace of scientific research on this topic in the United States did not gain much momentum until the 1980s. The impetus to seriously investigate late-life dementia, in part, reflected a growing awareness of the increasing demands on the health care system that would be made by the rapidly expanding elderly population; pressure from the Alzheimer's Disease and Related Disorders Association (now called the Alzheimer's Association); and the development of new technologies to investigate the brain. Although recent research efforts have not yielded a cure for progressive cognitive loss, they have significantly expanded our understanding of the various causes of mental decline, sensitized the professional community to the need for rigorous evaluation of late life mental changes, and launched some service programs to provide support and help to older people with cognitive difficulties and their families.

Definitions of Cognitive Problems

As discussed in Chapter 1, *DSM-III-R* is a psychiatric manual that provides specific rules for making a diagnosis of currently recognized mental disorders. In defining cognitive deficits, *DSM-III-R* makes a distinction between an organic mental *syndrome* and an organic mental *disorder*. An organic mental syndrome is a group of characteristic problems ("signs and symptoms") the cause of which is not necessarily known. In contrast, an organic mental disorder is a specific mental syndrome the cause of which is known or can be assumed to be known with a good degree of confidence. Since the cause or causes of cognitive problems are not often initially known, this distinction between a syndrome and a disorder allows a mental health professional to accurately characterize cognitive difficulties without presuming a specific cause. The goal of a good diagnostic work-up is to move from a diagnosis of organic mental syndrome to the more specific diagnosis of organic mental disorder. Although there are a variety of organic mental syndromes and organic mental disorders, we will focus on those of most frequent concern to older adults.

ORGANIC MENTAL SYNDROMES

Two organic mental syndromes most often seen in older adults are dementia and delirium. Dementia refers to deficits in short- and long-term memory often accompanied by difficulties in thinking and judgment, personality changes, and other cognitive problems. Delirium involves problems with maintaining and shifting attention, logical thinking, and speech as well as other difficulties. People with delirium often appear confused. These syndromes are not exclusive of one another—that is, a person with dementia may also have delirium.

Delirium

The following is a summary of *DSM-III-R* rules that mental health professionals use to make a diagnosis of delirium.

1. The individual evidences a reduced ability to concentrate or maintain attention to things outside of him- or herself. In addition, the individual has difficulty in shifting attention from one topic to another.

2. Thinking is disorganized. This is evident in speech that is unfocused, not easily understood, or irrelevant.

3. At least two of the following must exist:

   Reduced consciousness. The person may find it hard to stay awake.

   Misperceptions, illusions, or hallucinations. That is, the individual's capacity to accurately perceive his or her surroundings via the sense organs is diminished.

   Increased or decreased physical activity or strong emotional reactions.

   Disorientation with respect to time, place, or person.

   Memory problems.

4. Difficulties develop over a relatively short period of time (for example, a few hours or days) and fluctuate in their presence or severity over the course of a day.

5. Either of the following must be present:

There is evidence that there is a specific organic reason (based on history of current difficulties, a physical examination, or laboratory results) for the problem.

If there is no such evidence, an organic cause can be reasonably presumed if a nonorganic factor (such as another psychiatric disorder) is not the cause of the problem.

Dementia

Although the complete *DSM-III-R* criteria for this disorder and others that are discussed in this book are reprinted (with permission) in Appendix B, the following is a general summary of the rules for diagnosing dementia.

1. The individual must show impairment in short-term and long-term memory. Problems with short-term memory are in part determined by the mental health professional's naming three objects (for example, a watch, a ball, and a comb) and then asking the person being evaluated to recall the objects five minutes later. Long-term memory is evaluated by asking the individual to provide personal information that is normally well retained (for example, What are the names of your children? How old are you?) or common factual information (for example, Who is the current president of the United States?).

2. At least one of the following problems must be present:

Difficulties in abstract thinking. For example, the individual may not be able to define similarities or differences among a variety of objects or words.

Impaired judgment. This difficulty is most evident in an inability to reasonably deal with life issues (for example, interpersonal issues with family, friends, or work).

Other problems. These include an inability to use or understand words (aphasia), an inability to recognize familiar objects (agnosia), problems in physically manipulating things (apraxia), and problems with copying and drawing (constructional difficulties).

Personality changes. New personality characteristics may appear or there may be an accentuation of previous personality characteristics.

3. The problems in 1 and 2 are severe enough that they interfere with the individual's work, activities, or social relationships.

4. The individual was not in an episode of delirium when the above difficulties were present.

5. Either of these must be true:

The problem(s) being presented by the individual can be linked to an organic problem (for example, a biochemical disturbance).

If an organic factor cannot be identified as the cause of cognitive losses, the loss cannot be linked to any other nonorganic problem. For example, cognitive impairments might be present because the individual is seriously depressed.

The diagnosis of dementia is also rated according to its severity: mild, moderate, or severe.

ORGANIC MENTAL DISORDERS

There are a variety of known causes of dementia. Two of the most common types of dementia are primary degenerative dementia of the Alzheimer type (usually referred to as Alzheimer's disease) and multi-infarct dementia. The cause of Alzheimer's disease is not presently known. The cause of multi-infarct dementia is a series of small strokes (infarcts) that damage brain tissue over time. Additional causes of dementia include Parkinson's disease, chronic alcoholism, Pick's disease, and Creutzfeldt-Jakob disease. Conditions that cause dementia will be discussed in more detail later. The following are *DSM-III-R* criteria for the diagnosis of specific organic mental disorders.

Primary Degenerative Dementia of the Alzheimer Type

1. A dementia syndrome, as defined earlier, is present.

2. The dementia has an insidious onset (that is, it begins slowly and subtly and, at first, escapes notice) and is accompanied by progressive deterioration of the individual's abilities.

3. All other possible causes of dementia have been eliminated.

This condition is further characterized on the basis of whether it began before age 65 (presenile onset) or after age 65 (senile onset) and whether it is accompanied by delirium, delusions, depression, or none of these (referred to as uncomplicated Alzheimer's).

Multi-Infarct Dementia (MID)

1. A dementia syndrome, as defined earlier, is present.

2. Multi-infarct dementia (MID) is caused by a series of small strokes that progressively damage the brain. Although the person with MID may not be aware of these strokes, others may notice that he or she appears to be losing different mental abilities one step at a time. This is referred to as a step-wise deteriorating course. Since the area of the brain in which the small stroke or strokes occurs corresponds to the mental ability that is damaged, some abilities will remain unaffected while others will be impaired. This pattern of cognitive losses is sometimes referred to as the patchy distribution of deficits.

3. Certain neurological difficulties are present.

4. There is evidence of disease involving blood vessels in the brain (cerebrovascular disease) that is likely related to the individual's condition and that is

confirmed by personal history or medical tests (for example, a brain scan).

Two other categories of organic mental disorders are also sometimes used in the diagnosis of cognitive loss in older adults. "Senile dementia not otherwise specified" and "presenile dementia not otherwise specified" are categories reserved for, respectively, dementias that begin after age 65 or before age 65 and that cannot be classified by any other *DSM-III-R* dementia diagnosis. There are other dementias and delirium caused by drug or alcohol use that can also be diagnosed by *DSM-III-R*, as well as conditions caused by physical illnesses (e.g., brain tumor).

Frequency of Dementias and Delirium among Older Adults

Dementia is almost exclusively a condition of later life. It is the only psychiatric condition for which people experience increased risk in old age. A number of researchers have surveyed community-residing older adults to determine the prevalence (or frequency) of mild and severe forms of dementia. Two problems with research that has investigated the prevalence of mild dementia are that there is no standard definition of mild dementia and that symptoms of early dementia may be difficult to detect. Not surprisingly, researchers have reported widely varying estimates of the prevalence of mild dementia, although studies tend to indicate that about 11 percent of older adults have mild dementia. Until recently there was some general consensus on the prevalence of severe dementia, which was estimated to affect about 4 percent of people 65 or older. However, a very recent study in the Boston area suggests that the figure may be much higher, with perhaps as many as 10 percent of people over age 65 having Alzheimer's disease (in addition to those who have other forms of dementia). In nursing homes the prevalence of significant cognitive impairment is high—estimates range from 50–75 percent. Risk for dementia increases with age. Until recently it was believed that among persons 80 years or older the prevalence of dementia was about 20 percent. In contrast, recent research from the Boston-area study suggests that among persons 85 or older almost half show evidence of Alzheimer's disease (again, in addition to those with other forms of dementia).

Scientists are presently trying to integrate the Boston-area research into a larger body of previous scientific findings.

Alzheimer's disease is by far the most common cause of dementia. About 60 percent of dementias in people over age 65 are caused by Alzheimer's disease. The next most common form is multi-infarct dementia, which accounts for 10–20 percent of cases. Remaining cases of dementia are caused by a combination of Alzheimer's disease and multi-infarct dementia (known as mixed dementia); by rarer illnesses such as Pick's disease and Creutzfeldt-Jakob disease; by cognitive problems resulting from Parkinson's disease; and by conditions that are remediable or partially remediable including brain tumors and cognitive problems caused by medications, infection, malnutrition, alcohol, metabolic disturbances, or depression. Some mental health professionals have suggested that 10–20 percent of dementias may have remediable aspects. The frequency of delirium in older adults is not well known.

Causes of Delirium and Dementias

As has been discussed, delirium and dementias are clinical syndromes that can be caused by a variety of disorders. They may also coexist with one another. These conditions may be difficult to diagnose, particularly if the mental health professional is unfamiliar with cognitive and emotional disorders of late life.

DELIRIUM

As noted, delirium is a condition in which the individual has, among a variety of other problems, significant difficulties with concentrating, thinking logically, and speaking coherently. Delirium has been generally characterized as a disorder of attention. For example, it is difficult for a person with delirium to maintain a normal conversation without getting distracted. The individual loses the train of conversation and may switch from topic to topic for no apparent reason. Hallucinations and delusions may accompany delirium in addition to extreme emotional responses including anger, anxiety, fear, euphoria, and depression. Delirium usually comes on fairly suddenly and may last from a few hours to several weeks. Rarely does delirium persist longer than a month.

There are many possible causes of delirium. The major causes include the following.

Intoxication from prescribed drugs or from interactions among drugs.

Metabolic disturbances. That is, there is a disruption of the complex physical and chemical processes that sustain life.

Cardiovascular problems (difficulties involving the heart and blood vessels).

Infection, fever, or both.

Reactions to alcohol.

Pain.

Anemia (a deficiency of certain components of the blood).

Tumors.

Brain disorders.

Chronic lung disease.

Reaction to hospitalization.

Common to this wide variety of causes of delirium is disruption of normal functioning of the brain.

DEMENTIAS

Irreversible Dementias

As discussed, dementia involves problems in short- and long-term memory that are often accompanied by difficulties in thinking and judgment and by personality changes. Diagnosis of a dementia *syndrome* should lead the mental health professional to search for the disorder causing the syndrome. Some dementias are reversible—that is, there may be drug, metabolic, psychiatric, or other problems that when remedied result in disappearance of the dementia syndrome. Most dementias are not reversible—the cause is a permanent defect in the brain. The causes of those defects are the subject of a fair amount of current research.

ALZHEIMER'S DISEASE   Alzheimer's disease is the cause of the dementia disorder that bears its name. Although it is the most common of the dementias, the cause or causes of Alzheimer's disease are not understood. There are, however, a variety of genetic, viral, environmental, immunological, and other theories about the cause of Alzheimer's disease. Two things are known: (1) Alzheimer's disease is associated with characteristic microscopic brain changes that may be seen when the brain is autopsied, and (2) people with Alzheimer's disease have decreased amounts of choline acetyltransferase, a chemical in the brain that plays an important role in human learning and memory.

One theory currently being researched is that Alzheimer's is a genetically transmitted disease. An intriguing piece of evidence that provided an impetus to research possible genetic factors in Alzheimer's disease came from observations of people with Down's syndrome. In middle age, people with Down's syndrome (a genetic abnormality that results in varying degrees of mental retardation) develop a type of dementia that is remarkably similar to Alzheimer's disease. In addition, the incidence of Down's syndrome may be higher in the families of people with Alzheimer's disease than in the population at large. Other studies have found that the risk of Alzheimer's disease is higher in relatives of some persons with Alzheimer's disease than it is in other people. At this point, it appears that the earlier Alzheimer's disease strikes an individual, the greater the risk that family members of that individual will also develop Alzheimer's disease in later life. It is difficult, however, to confidently predict the degree of that risk.

One of the difficulties of doing research on the possible genetic determinants of Alzheimer's disease is that the illness appears so late in life. Scientists studying the frequency of Alzheimer's disease in a particular family may not detect the disease in some individuals either because those individuals died of other illnesses (but would have acquired Alzheimer's disease if they had lived longer) or because, at the time of the study, those individuals did not evidence Alzheimer's disease (but will evidence it when they are much older). Recent studies of older adults who are identical twins have found that one twin may evidence Alzheimer's disease while the other does not. This suggests, among other things, that there may be factors other than genetic ones that are related to the onset of Alzheimer's disease. The question of the familial risk of Alzheimer's disease is, of course, a very important one for family members of people with this disorder. At this point, however, scientists can only conclude that there may be additional risk for family members of Alzheimer's disease patients. Recently researchers have reported the possible location of a gene associated with some kinds of Alzheimer's disease, but this is only a first step in understanding the genetic underpinnings of this illness.

In principle, there may be increased risk in the family members of some Alzheimer's disease patients for reasons that may not be genetic but environmental. Some scientists have suggested that Alzheimer's disease may be virally caused. One incentive to study possible viral causes of Alzheimer's disease comes from research on the disease kuru. Kuru, a neurological disorder that eventually results in dementia, was documented in certain tribes, predominantly among women, who reside only in the highlands of New Guinea. For many years the reasons for the disease were unknown. Eventually anthropologists discovered that tribes with a high prevalence of kuru practiced cannibalism in which the brains were eaten by women of the tribe and the rest of the body was eaten by the men. The possibility that kuru was transmitted by a virus received support when scientists injected brain tissue from a kuru victim into a chimpanzee and the animal eventually developed the disease. The period of time from infection to the development of symptoms in the chimpanzee was several years, which led scientists to conclude that this virus was of the "slow" variety—that is, symptoms only appear a considerable length of time after infection. Acquired immune deficiency syndrome (AIDS) is, for example, a slow virus. However, efforts to try to transmit Alzheimer's disease from humans to primates have not met with success.

Another possible cause of Alzheimer's disease that has been examined is aluminum. Some researchers have found high levels of aluminum in the brains of Alzheimer's disease patients. Other researchers found that when experimental animals were given large amounts of aluminum they showed microscopic brain changes similar to those found in Alzheimer's disease patients. Later scientific work, however, failed to confirm the earlier findings. In addition, the brain changes seen in experimental animals exposed to toxic amounts of aluminum are in actuality somewhat different from those documented in Alzheimer's disease patients. At present, many members of the scientific community feel is it unlikely that Alzheimer's disease is caused by excess consumption of aluminum.

There are additional theories. Some researchers have reported abnormalities in the immune systems of Alzheimer's disease patients. This has led to speculation that immunological problems might be a cause of the illness. It is not clear, however, whether immunological irregularities among Alzheimer's disease victims are the cause or consequence of the disease. Another idea is that Alzheimer's disease might be the result of accumulated damages ("insults") to the brain from various sources. Some have suggested that a combination of factors results in Alzheimer's disease. Important basic research on the possible origins of Alzheimer's disease continues, and we can anticipate further scientific clues regarding its cause or causes in the coming decade.

MULTI-INFARCT DEMENTIA   The second most common type of dementia is multi-infarct dementia. Multi-infarct dementia is the progressive loss of brain tissue through a series of small strokes (infarcts) caused by occlusions, or blockages, of arteries to the brain. These strokes are so small that the individual may not be aware of them when they happen. Symptoms depend on the location of the infarct. After each infarct or series of infarcts the individual may lose another perceptible level of mental abilities. As the damage from the infarcts accumulates, the individual shows more widespread evidence of diminished mental ability. Over the course of years, patients afflicted with Alzheimer's disease and multi-infarct dementia may both evidence broad mental deficits that are difficult to distinguish from one another. Whereas the onset of Alzheimer's disease is typically after age 65, the beginning of multi-infarct dementia is usually between the ages of 40 and 60.

Risk factors for multi-infarct dementia are those that are typically associated with cardiac disease and stroke. These include high levels of cholesterol, smoking, and high blood pressure.

OTHER IRREVERSIBLE AND PROGRESSIVE DEMENTIAS   There are also other, much less common causes of dementia. Like Alzheimer's disease and multi-infarct dementia, some of these dementias are irreversible and progressive—that is, they get worse over time.

Parkinson's disease is a neurological disorder in which the individual evidences physical rigidity, tremors (shaking), and difficulty walking. Parkinson's disease patients may also become demented. Parkinson's disease is caused by the deficiency of a critical brain substance, the neurotransmitter dopamine. Fortunately, physical symptoms can be treated fairly effectively in many patients in the early years of the illness with the drug L-Dopa. L-Dopa does not, however, appear to improve cognitive problems. The illness may affect as many as one-quarter million Americans, most of them older adults. It is thought that at least one-third of people with Parkinson's disease will eventually develop a dementia syndrome.

As noted earlier, the disease kuru is a virally transmitted type of dementia that is found in New Guinea. A related disorder is Creutzfeldt-Jakob disease, which also has been shown to be virally transmitted in laboratory animals. General paresis, a dementing condition caused by neurosyphilis, is a sexually transmitted bacterial infection that was seen much more frequently before the advent of antibiotics. Pick's disease, another cause of irreversible dementia, is a very rare condition that usually appears between the ages of 40 and 60. Some authors have suggested that the condition may have an important genetic component. Pick's disease is similar in its symptoms to Alzheimer's disease, and even astute mental health professionals may not be able to distinguish it from Alzheimer's disease. Some researchers have reported that personality changes are the most evident symptom at the beginning of Pick's disease and that only later do memory problems and associated difficulties appear. Other rare conditions that cause dementia include Huntington's disease and Wilson's disease.

Nonprogressive Dementias

While most dementias tend to worsen over time, some do not. Nonprogressive dementias are usually caused by brain injuries and typically only affect certain abilities. The most common types of nonprogressive dementias result from strokes, trauma to the head, and aneurysms (weakening and eventual breakage of an artery within the brain). Determining whether symptoms of cognitive impairment are progressive or nonprogressive is critical because the long-range implications of the two types are very different. For example, planning for the future of a person with a progressive dementia is quite different from planning for the future of an individual with a circumscribed loss of abilities that will not worsen.

Reversible Dementias

As with delirium, there are dementia syndromes caused by factors that might be reversible. These include drugs and alcohol, nutritional deficiencies, tumors, infections, metabolic disturbances, endocrine disturbances, brain disorders, psychiatric difficulties, and neurological problems. Considerable effort in the diagnostic process, in fact, is devoted to determining whether the patient's cognitive problems are a result of remediable causes. One of the most common causes of reversible dementia is prescribed drugs. Certain drugs or combinations of drugs may affect brain functioning in a way that causes a dementia syndrome. Lifelong alcoholism or the onset of alcoholism in late life may yield cognitive changes consistent with a dementia syndrome. A deficiency in vitamin B-12, folic acid, niacin, or other deficiencies may also cause dementia.

Normal pressure hydrocephalus (NPH) is a condition that when corrected can result in considerable reduction of dementia symptoms. NPH results from obstruction of the movement of cerebrospinal fluid. The condition is not readily detected because measures of pressure within the brain register as normal. However, other medical tests can be used to diagnose NPH. The problem is treated by placing a shunt in the brain that drains off excess fluid. This surgical procedure appears to be successful in about half of the cases. Tumors of the brain or metastases to the brain from cancers elsewhere in the body may result in dementia that, in some cases, may recede when the tumor(s) or the condition causing it is treated. Brain infections may also be associated with dementia. In the case of neurosyphilis, treatment of the condition may prevent the onset of dementia. Endocrine abnormalities, most notably thyroid gland dysfunction, can cause cognitive difficulties. Early treatment of this medical problem is important since, if left untreated, it may result in irreversible cognitive loss.

As discussed in Chapter 1, depression may be accompanied by cognitive changes that appear similar to dementia. The term *pseudodementia* and others have been used to describe this phenomenon. Symptoms of depression and cognitive loss may be evident in both clinical depression and the dementia syndrome; it is therefore sometimes difficult to distinguish between the two. To add to the challenge of making an accurate diagnosis, both may exist at the same time. Persons experiencing cognitive impairment that is secondary to depression will usually have a history of depression, report an abrupt onset of cognitive difficulties, have cognitive losses that are milder than those seen in patients with progressive dementia, and have cognitive problems that are selective rather than global. In addition, some researchers have reported that dementia patients will tend to disguise their cognitive problems whereas individuals with pseudodementia will openly complain of their memory difficulties.

Evaluation of Cognitive Problems

As should be clear from the preceding discussion, the diagnosis of cognitive difficulties in the older adult involves consideration of a wide variety of both apparent and less obvious factors. Unfortunately, several studies have found that errors in the diagnosis of dementia are not uncommon, particularly by physicians without any psychiatric training. Diagnostic inaccuracy is primarily a function of some health professionals' lack of up-to-date knowledge about the diagnosis of cognitive problems. Ideally, the diagnostic evaluation of cognitive problems is a multistage process that usually includes: (1) determining the nature of current difficulties, (2) obtaining a history of current and past related difficulties, (3) assessing current cognitive abilities, (4) determining whether psychiatrically associated problems exist, (5) conducting a medical evaluation, (6) evaluating the individual's ability to function on a day-to-day basis, and (7) evaluating the breadth and quality of the older adult's social relationships and environmental resources.

DETERMINING THE NATURE OF CURRENT DIFFICULTIES

The first step in a diagnostic evaluation is to conduct a thorough assessment of those difficulties that motivated the older adult to seek an evaluation. Commonly, however, the family has brought the individual for an evaluation. Since cognitive problems often result in impaired judgment, it is usually at the urging of others that persons with dementia or delirium are evaluated. As will be discussed at more length later, the families of dementia patients typically play a critical role in providing care for them.

The initial diagnostic interview with the older adult will usually include an interview with him or her as well as an interview with a key informant—that is, an individual, usually a family member, who can provide additional or clarifying information. Since the psychiatric diagnostic system in *DSM-III-R* only offers broad guidelines regarding symptoms that must be present for a diagnosis of dementia or delirium, the clinical judgment of the mental health professional about whether a particular symptom is severe or significant enough to be counted toward the diagnosis is crucial. The need to ask clear and specific questions about the older adult's concerns is important since individuals share widely varying notions of what constitutes, for example, memory loss, confusion, or other symptoms.

> Gloria Barnard was evaluated at the geriatric mental health clinic because of her fear that she had "Alzheimer's disease." Mrs. Barnard, a well-educated woman, complained of her "failing memory" and "problems with concentration." "Frankly, Doctor," Mrs. Barnard confessed, "I'm afraid to get the bad news about my mental capacities—but I'm prepared." A careful evaluation of Mrs. Barnard's concerns revealed that her appraisal of a "failing memory" was based on her present inability to remember the telephone numbers of all of her friends as she had been able to throughout most of her life. Her perception that she had "problems with concentration" was based on the fact that she no longer read the *New York Times* from cover to cover each day. When told that she had no evidence of Alzheimer's disease or any other dementia, Mrs. Barnard was greatly relieved and wondered whether she had seen "too many programs on television about Alzheimer's disease."

As per *DSM-III-R* criteria, memory loss will be of key interest in making a diagnosis of a dementia syndrome, as will other difficulties including impairment of abstract thinking, judgment, and language and personality changes. Attentional difficulties will be most important in making a diagnosis of delirium, along with other possible symptoms including disorganized thinking; problems with staying awake; misperceptions, illusions, or hallucinations; altered levels of physical activity or emotional responsivity; disorientation; and memory problems. Sensitive and thoughtful questioning of the patient and the family will usually elicit enough information for the clinician to make a reasoned diagnosis after the complete diagnostic process is completed.

OBTAINING A HISTORY OF CURRENT AND PAST RELATED DIFFICULTIES

An integral part of the initial examination is finding out when the current difficulties began. Most people with Alzheimer's disease have a slow (sometimes called insidious) onset of difficulties. That is, the condition may have existed in a milder form for some time, but only when the older adult had significant difficulties were prior problems recognized. A family member may note in retrospect, for example, that the older adult evidenced increasing difficulty with remembering appointments, names of newly met individuals, or the placement of household items. Multi-infarct dementia, on the other hand, is caused by a series of small strokes that usually result in observable losses of select abilities. For example, an individual may be observed to have developed problems with finding the right words (a form of aphasia) within a relatively short period of time. Delirium and reversible dementias may come on suddenly. For persons with dementia symptoms that are secondary to depression (so-called pseudodementia), the onset of symptoms will in part depend on the type of depression from which the individual is suffering. For persons with discrete episodes of depression, as often found in major depression, the onset of symptoms may appear more abruptly than if the individual has a chronic depression such as dysthymia.

ASSESSING CURRENT COGNITIVE ABILITIES

One of the most common objective ways to assess an individual's current cognitive functioning is with a mental status test. A mental status test is typically a brief series of questions from which the mental health professional can obtain a rough estimate of the severity of cognitive impairment. The questions contained in these tests cover well-known information such as, "What day is this?" "Where are you?" and "Who is the current president of the United States?" Mental status tests may also include, for example, requests that the older adult follow simple instructions, draw a figure, or make basic calculations. A major advantage of mental status tests is that the content is basic enough so that errors provide a strong clue for the presence of clinically significant cognitive problems. A disadvantage of these tests is that they may not be sensitive to more subtle cognitive problems. It is important to emphasize, however, that errors on mental status tests are only one piece of evidence in a larger diagnostic puzzle.

More detailed assessment of an individual's cognitive difficulties can be done with neuropsychological testing. A wide variety of tests of cognitive functions has been developed by neuropsychologists. As noted earlier, neuropsychologists are psychologists who specialize in the measurement of specific brain functions. A mental health professional might request neuropsychological testing of a broad range of abilities or only of specific areas of concern. Usually neuropsychological testing will be conducted when, after initial evaluation, it is still unclear whether the older adult has a dementia and additional evidence is needed. On the other hand, sometimes it is clear that the adult person has a dementia syndrome, but the mental health professional desires to identify which mental capacities are impaired and to what degree they are affected. This information can be valuable in deciding which activities the individual may or may not be capable of performing. The information can also be utilized as a baseline against which to judge future cognitive deterioration among those with progressive dementias.

DETERMINING WHETHER PSYCHIATRICALLY ASSOCIATED PROBLEMS EXIST

Psychiatrically related problems such as depression, delusions, and hallucinations need to be evaluated. Initially, depression needs to be assessed as a possible cause of cognitive problems. As has been discussed at some length, depression may be accompanied by cognitive deficits that, at first, seem to be evidence of an irreversible dementia. On the other hand, dementia may be accompanied by depression that is a reaction to the loss of mental abilities. As will be detailed later, treatment of depression in a person with dementia may improve not only the individual's emotional well-being but also, to some extent, the individual's cognitive abilities.

Other psychiatrically related difficulties that should be evaluated include delusions and hallucinations. Delusions typically occur in demented patients when the individual, presumably trying to compensate for problems caused by memory loss, develops false beliefs to make sense of certain experiences. For example, an older woman may forget where she placed her wedding ring and, as a result, become convinced that someone entered her home and took it. Less commonly, an individual with dementia may experience hallucinations—false sensory perceptions such as seeing or hearing things that are not present. The presence of delusions or hallucinations in an older adult with cognitive problems may also be associated with delirium.

The mental health professional must consider, however, whether the presence of delusions or hallucinations might be a result of other disorders. For example, persons with delusional disorder may hold false beliefs that are unrelated to cognitive impairment. Persons with schizophrenia usually have psychotic episodes and may experience delusions, hallucinations, or other symptoms. In brief, other psychiatric problems must be considered as a possible cause of certain symptoms.

CONDUCTING A MEDICAL EVALUATION

A medical examination should always be conducted on an older adult who appears to have delirium or dementia. A medical examination should also be done if an individual previously diagnosed with dementia takes a sudden turn for the worse. The primary purpose of a medical evaluation is to investigate whether any number of different medical conditions might be the cause of cognitive problems. Blood tests, a chest X-ray, an electrocardiogram, and other tests are typically obtained. A CT (computerized axial transverse tomography) scan, in which multiple X-ray pictures of the brain are taken, is recommended. Although certain specific changes are often seen in dementia (most notably atrophy of the brain), such changes are also sometimes seen in older adults who are not demented. The CT scan is therefore not a definitive test for dementia. CT scans are most useful, however, in documenting the presence of brain tumors that may be operable. Other tests may also be done at the discretion of the medical doctor. A medical/neurological evaluation may aid in identifying whether the older person has cerebrovascular problems that are associated with multi-infarct dementia. A medical examination also plays a critical role in the evaluation of delirium, which, if untreated, in some cases may be life threatening.

Efforts are under way to see if it might be possible to develop a more definitive test for Alzheimer's disease. As noted, at present the only definitive test is evaluation of the patient's brain at autopsy. Some researchers are currently exploring whether there might be certain characteristic chemical "markers" of Alzheimer's disease that might be present in, for example, the patient's cerebrospinal fluid. At present, however, no such test is available for clinical use.

EVALUATING THE INDIVIDUAL'S ABILITY TO FUNCTION

At the beginning of the diagnostic process, it is useful for the mental health professional to make a general appraisal of the older adult's ability to carry on the day-to-day activities that are necessary to live independently. Since individuals with dementia vary considerably in their functional abilities, detailed questioning is important. For example, to what degree is the older person able to carry out rudimentary aspects of daily living such as eating, toileting, dressing, and bathing? Is the individual able to carry on more complicated tasks such as shopping, cooking, cleaning, using a telephone, and using transportation? With regard to transportation, is the older individual driving? If so, does this present a danger either to him- or herself or to others? It is also useful to inquire about daily activities like paying bills, making appointments, and negotiating with tradespersons. The family or close friends are usually the best source of this information.

EVALUATING THE SOCIAL AND PHYSICAL ENVIRONMENT

The breadth and quality of social relationships available to a person with dementia make a critical difference in the quality of life he or she will live. These relationships may also determine whether the person lives at home or in an institution. The mental health professional must ask him- or herself: Who is the primary caregiver who provides the most help to the older person? What degree of commitment exists to provide care now and in the future? Is this individual aware of financial, recreational, and social services available in the community? Does the primary caregiver appear emotionally overtaxed as a result of caregiving responsibilities? Are other persons available to provide help to the primary caregiver? What is their degree of commitment to care? Does the older individual have friends with whom regular contact is maintained? If not, why not? Has the older individual maintained activities in which he or she participated before the onset of dementia? If not, why not? Has the older individual unnecessarily stopped activities in which he or she is still capable of participating? On the other hand, does participation exceed existing capabilities?

An assessment of the older person's physical environment may be beneficial. A home visit may yield additional clues to the individual's capacity to function on a day-to-day basis. Such a visit may also help to identify environmental circumstances that may be harmful. Some demented older persons may, for example, place themselves and others in danger by having easy access to stoves, which, because of memory problems, may be left on. In reality, few mental health professionals make such home assessments. However, a general inquiry about some of these issues may yield some important clues to any environmental problems.

When the diagnostic process is complete, the results need to be communicated sensitively and clearly to family members involved with the patient. In most instances family members are very distressed at this point and may fear the worst. Given the fairly extensive media coverage of Alzheimer's disease in recent years, for many people Alzheimer's disease *is* their worst fear. Unfortunately, not all health professionals make the necessary efforts to judge the psychological impact of diagnostic information that is communicated to the family.

Sylvia Snow brought her 58-year-old husband, Dennis, to the geriatric mental health clinic because he was no longer able to work as an accountant due to significant problems with memory. She said that her husband had been evaluated by a medical doctor a few months earlier but she was not clear what the outcome of the evaluation had been. She did say, however, that she had been told by the doctor's nurse over the telephone that her husband had "primary degenerative dementia." "I was relieved to hear this," said Mrs. Snow. "At least it wasn't Alzheimer's disease or something like that."

Susan Joseph, the daughter of an older man who was diagnosed with Alzheimer's disease by a prominent local neurologist, came to the geriatric mental health clinic because of deep emotional distress related to her father's diagnosis. Ms. Joseph reported that, after a thorough evaluation of her father, the doctor had met with the two of them. "Yup, he's got Alzheimer's disease all right. Better take the trip around the world you always wanted, Mr. Joseph, because in six months you'll be in pretty sad shape."

Treatment of Cognitive Problems

Treatment exists for some aspects of cognitive problems. In this section we will discuss two types of treatment strategies for cognitive difficulties: (1) medical and pharmacologic, and (2) psychosocial interventions to help older adults with dementia and their families. Medical treatments usually play a central role in helping people with delirium or reversible dementias. Pharmacologic treatments are often utilized to help reduce the behavioral and emotional difficulties that usually accompany dementia. And several drugs have been or are currently being investigated to see if they might slow the dementia process. Psychosocial interventions are available to assist the patient and family to better cope with dementia.

MEDICAL AND PHARMACOLOGICAL TREATMENTS

Delirium and Reversible Dementias

As discussed earlier, delirium is a condition characterized by confusion and other difficulties caused by one or more underlying problems that if identified and treated can stop the delirium.

Finding and treating the cause of delirium is critical since some cases, if left untreated, will progress to dementia or even death. Common causes of delirium are medication side effects (usually from psychiatric drugs like sleeping pills or drugs for high blood pressure) and endocrine problems (most commonly hypothyroidism, a condition characterized by an underactive thyroid). Reducing or stopping medications or remedying underlying medical conditions is the usual way to treat delirium.

> Claudia Parrish woke her husband earlier than usual. "There are elephants outside the window," she exclaimed, "and last night I saw little girls in colorful dresses in the bathroom." Thinking that his wife was joking, Mr. Parrish went back to sleep. When he awoke later he found his wife in the kitchen talking nonsensibly. He telephoned the family doctor, who erroneously said that Mrs. Parrish probably suffered from "Alzheimer's disease." Dissatisfied with this assessment, Mr. Parrish took his wife to a psychiatrist, who after a careful evaluation determined that Mrs. Parrish was suffering from delirium. He told Mr. Parrish to stop all medications that his wife was taking—and within a few days the hallucinations stopped. Mr. Parrish later discovered that, unknown to him, his wife had been taking a large variety of prescribed and nonprescribed medications, some of which she had "borrowed" from friends because they found the drugs "helpful."

Treatment approaches are similar for people with reversible dementias (i.e., identifying underlying medical problems or medication-induced symptoms). Dementia symptoms caused by depression (i.e., so-called pseudodementia) are usually treated by prescribing antidepressant medication. If the older adult indeed has pseudodementia, the cognitive deficits will usually clear after adequate treatment with antidepressant medications.

Irreversible Dementias

Multi-infarct dementia, a disease of the cerebrovascular system, is usually treated with aspirin and anti-clotting drugs with the intent of possibly slowing the progress of this illness. Little research has documented to what degree this treatment is helpful.

Other existing treatments for cognitive impairment are, for the most part, experimental. Most of these have been directed to the treatment of Alzheimer's disease. It is important to emphasize at the outset, however, that none of these treatments has been found to have a significant effect on irreversible dementia.

One group of compounds used to try to improve the cognitive abilities of people with dementia are stimulants. Stimulants activate the central nervous system. They have specifically been evaluated for their possible role in enhancing attention and performance. Examples of stimulant drugs are methylphenidate, amphetamines, pentylenetetrazol, and pipradrol. Carefully designed studies have not, however, found any significant improvement in cognitive abilities from these drugs. Other compounds called vasodilators are designed to improve blood flow to the brain. Examples of these include papaverine, cyclandelate, and isoxsuprine. Again, research has not found any significant improvement in the condition of people with dementia from this type of medication. Another effort has been to enhance brain metabolism. Although the drug Hydergine was at first thought to be a vasodilator, some now believe that it primarily acts to enhance brain metabolism. Studies have found that Hydergine is associated with modest improvement in some aspects of mental and emotional functioning in some dementia patients. The medication may be most effective for individuals with milder forms of dementia.

Given evidence that Alzheimer's disease is associated with disturbance of the cholinergic system in the brain, the major experimental drug strategy has been to try to enhance the functioning of this system. Among a variety of compounds that have been investigated, only physostigmine has resulted in some detectable, though far from dramatic, improvement in the cognitive functioning of some individuals. Recently another compound designed to enhance the cholinergic system, tetrahydroaminoacridine (THA or Tacrine) was reported to have resulted in dramatic improvement in a small number of patients. Some researchers have expressed caution about this early research on THA and believe that more extensive studies of the drug are needed. Such studies are now ongoing. Other drugs are also currently under investigation, including the hormones adrenocorticotropic hormone (ACTH) and vasopressin (Vp), L-Dopa (often used in the treatment of Parkinson's disease), and enkephalins (brain substances involved in the mediation of pain). Some of these drugs have shown some very limited usefulness in improving select cognitive abilities in dementia patients. Despite the limited success of the above treatments, hope remains that some form of treatment for dementia will be found within the next decade.

Different stages of dementing illness are often accompanied by behavioral or emotional difficulties that may be treated with psychiatric medications. In the early stages of dementia, 20–25 percent of patients may experience some form of depression. This is believed to be largely an emotional reaction, a consequence of the older adult's awareness of his or her declining mental abilities. Tricyclic antidepressants or MAO inhibitors are sometimes prescribed. As discussed in Chapter 1, physicians prescribing these medications must take into account age-related differences in the way that older people metabolize drugs. Some psychiatrists have found that antidepressant treatment is most effective for individuals in the earlier stages of dementia. In contrast, antidepressant treatment of older adults with more advanced cases of the illness may create agitation and confusion; hence, one should be very cautious when prescribing antidepressants to persons in the later stages of dementia.

Individuals with more advanced dementia may be prone to disturbances of sleep, confusion, paranoid thoughts, periods of crying or anger, assaultive behavior, and other difficulties. Benzodiazepines, a type of anti-anxiety medication, or neuroleptics, major tranquilizers primarily used in the treatment of schizophrenia, may be prescribed. There is some concern about possible consequences of prescribing these drugs, especially neuroleptics, in older people. First, despite the fact that neuroleptics are often prescribed to older people with dementia (particularly those residing in nursing homes), few research studies have clearly documented that the medications are helpful. Second, longer-term exposure to neuroleptics is associated with a possibly permanent side effect called tardive dyskinesia (TD), which is primarily characterized by involuntary muscle movements. Recent research has shown that even brief exposure to neuroleptics in older individuals may prompt TD symptoms. Third, treatment with benzodiazepines or neuroleptics that is not carefully monitored may result in delirium or even aggravation of dementia. Fourth, some have argued that neuroleptic drugs are sometimes used to tranquilize dementia patients in lieu of efforts to solve environmental difficulties that may be precipitating symptoms of emotional or behavioral distress. Most would agree that prescribing neuroleptics to older people with dementia must be done only after carefully evaluating symptoms and weighing the possible benefits and potential costs of this type of medication.

In the most advanced stages of dementia, individuals may show severe behavioral and cognitive problems and often are placed in residential institutions like nursing homes. Advanced dementia patients may sometimes be very withdrawn and appear lifeless; at other times they may scream, assault others, and wander aimlessly. Neuroleptic medications are often prescribed for persons with these symptoms. Other medications also have been tried for uncontrollable behavior, including lithium and propranolol. As with neuroleptics, little research has been done to investigate the efficacy of these medications for dementia patients.

PSYCHO-SOCIAL TREATMENTS

Individual Treatment of the Older Adult

As noted, some individuals in the earlier stages of dementia may become depressed because of the realization that their mental abilities are declining. Some mental health professionals have found that supportive counseling to these persons may help to reduce anxiety and depression and promote better adaptation to dementia. This type of counseling involves allowing the older adult to express feelings of distress over the loss of cognitive abilities, providing emotional support and encouragement, and assisting the person to make realistic plans for the future. This type of supportive therapy is a delicate balance of acknowledging the existence of a serious problem while trying to create some degree of hopefulness in the individual. This may be accomplished in part by offering the older adult alternate ways of thinking about living with chronic illness that promote more adaptive coping. For example, the older adult's perception that dementia is an affliction over which he or she has no control may be reframed so that dementia is instead viewed as a challenge that can be met by utilizing all personal and familial resources that the individual has carefully developed throughout his or her lifetime.

Eleanor Wall came for a mental health evaluation shortly after she retired as a high school teacher. She retired in large part because of increasing forgetfulness and a realization that she was having difficulty remembering from day to day what she had taught in her classes. She also complained of getting lost while driving on two occasions and of some difficulty finding words to express herself.

Mrs. Wall experienced a deep sense of loss upon her retirement from a career to which she had devoted her life as well as upon the realization that her mental abilities were failing. She complained of intermittent depression, feelings of hopelessness, anxiety, and reduced interest in doing those things she normally enjoyed. Psychiatric and medical evaluations were conducted that suggested she was suffering from Alzheimer's disease. Neuropsychological testing found that she indeed suffered from significant memory problems, some word-finding difficulty, and visual-spatial problems. On the other hand, testing also revealed that Mrs. Wall had other mental abilities that were well preserved and that prior to her recent difficulties she had been an exceptionally intelligent individual.

Because of continuing feelings of depression, Mrs. Wall requested counseling, which she received for three months. At first Mrs. Wall expressed anxiety and fear over her memory loss, saying that she felt as though she was "falling into a bottomless pit from which I will never return." She found it useful to talk about her fears, which she had carefully concealed from her family to "protect them." She also expressed anger and blame toward herself for her declining mental abilities. Despite her lifelong intellectual prowess, Mrs. Wall had always harshly judged her mental abilities, and the onset of Alzheimer's disease only exacerbated this problem. The psychologist working with Mrs. Wall encouraged her to more realistically judge the limits of her responsibility for her current difficulties, to appreciate those abilities she continued to possess, and to make changes in her daily routine to reduce the impact of her memory loss. Mrs. Wall was very responsive to this supportive counseling and experienced a concurrent reduction in feelings of anxiety, depression, and hopelessness.

Family Focused Treatments

In the last ten years there has been considerable research and interest in understanding the difficulties faced by the caregivers of persons with dementia. A number of research studies have documented that family caregivers of dementia patients experience fairly high levels of depression, anxiety, and physical health problems. In large measure these physical and mental health problems are a result of the stresses associated with the care of a dementia patient. Dementia patients are typically cared for by spouses or adult children in their own homes. Despite the erroneous belief that older individuals are abandoned to nursing homes, most families are very reluctant to institutionalize the dementia patient unless it is absolutely necessary. Family members may literally devote many years of their lives to the care of a loved one.

Most caregiving family members face a host of responsibilities aptly described by the title of a popular book on this topic, *The 36-Hour Day*. The type of care for a person with dementia usually depends on the stage of the illness. At one point or another in the dementia process most caregivers will have to contend with the older adult's decreasing ability to care for him- or herself. At first it may be necessary to provide some additional assistance to the dementia patient in performing household responsibilities like shopping, cooking, and cleaning, but as the illness progresses it becomes necessary to help the person to dress, eat, and bathe. As noted, there may be psychiatrically associated difficulties like depression, delusions, or hallucinations or behavioral problems like wandering off, getting lost, or engaging in behaviors that put the older person and his or her family in danger (e.g., leaving the stove on).

Family caregivers must also seek information on existing social and medical resources and negotiate with the providers of those services. Financial difficulties sometimes confront family caregivers, particularly if it is necessary to hire a home health attendant to be with the demented individual. If the individual is placed in a nursing home, the financial costs can be enormous. Caring for a relative with dementia may create family strains. Some adult children of dementia patients complain of an inequitable distribution of caregiving responsibilities among the siblings or disagree with their siblings about which course of action is best. Some persons caring for individuals with dementia either do not have available or do not appropriately use informal (e.g., family and friends) or formal (e.g., day treatment programs) supports. These supports usually play an important role in helping to ease the practical and emotional burdens of caregiving. Without such supports, family caregivers run the risk of stress-related emotional and physical problems. And beyond these day-to-day practical demands there is the personal anguish of witnessing the mental deterioration of a beloved spouse or parent. Some family caregivers have described progressive dementia as the painful "loss of self."

Probably the most comprehensive approach to family care of the dementia patient has been developed by psychologist Steven Zarit and his colleagues. Dr. Zarit, one of the first mental health professionals to carefully document the emotional and practical difficulties faced by families caring for dementia patients, has developed a stress management model for support of caregivers to dementia patients. The aims of this program are to enhance the family member's ability to manage dementia-associated problems and to help him or her learn to use existing social resources. Individual counseling, family counseling, and support groups are usually part of this approach.

The first step in the stress management model is to evaluate the difficulties faced by and the resources of the family of a dementia patient. Treatment begins by providing information to the family about dementia, discussing available dementia treatments, explaining why the dementia patient may act in certain ways, and addressing other issues as well. An accurate understanding of dementing illness is the foundation on which more specific problem-solving efforts are built. Caregivers may not understand that the problems experienced by the older adult are a result of a brain disorder. For example, some families may view dementia as a "failure of will" on the part of the dementia sufferer. They may feel frustrated that their efforts to push the older adult to be more active or to think positively do not work.

> After Lois Allen was diagnosed with Alzheimer's disease, the psychologist decided to make a visit to her home. In part, the visit was prompted because her husband appeared to be particularly frustrated over Mrs. Allen's inability to function at home. When the psychologist arrived, he found a slightly bewildered Mrs. Allen seated at the kitchen table with an array of household objects, arithmetic flash cards, and paper and pencils spread in front of her. Mr. Allen explained that he had just finished his daily "lesson" with his wife and, as usual, she had performed miserably. Mr. Allen, a former high school teacher, explained that he had been trying to improve his wife's mind by a variety of "mind exercises" he had developed and that if his wife "really tried harder her mind would improve."

Some family members may misinterpret the reasons for or the meaning of things the dementia patient has done. For example, many dementia patients may ask the same question over and over. Some families feel that this is done deliberately to annoy them and that the patient could stop this if he or she wanted. In family-focused treatment caregivers are taught that the repetitive questions reflect efforts by the patient to try to remember and to understand things that have been forgotten—including the fact that the same question may have been asked only minutes before. Some dementia patients may accuse family members of stealing things, which may be misinterpreted as a deliberate attempt to hurt or humiliate the family member. The family will be told that this behavior is an effort by the dementia patient to make sense of why things cannot be found. In large measure, steps are taken to help the family to reinterpret the dementia patient's behavior in light of the facts of dementing illness.

The next stage of this family-oriented treatment is to teach certain problem-solving skills. The mental health professional will work with the family member to identify specific problems, generate a variety of possible solutions, try out chosen solutions, and evaluate the usefulness of each solution. If a particular solution is not effective, other solutions are tried. A similar problem-solving approach is applied to helping caregivers to fully utilize other family members, friends, and neighbors in obtaining practical and emotional support. Caregivers are also taught how to better use existing formal supports like community agencies. Family members participating in such programs usually express enthusiasm about them, although research so far has shown the programs to have only circumscribed effects on improving the emotional adjustment of caregivers who participate.

Other approaches exist. One program teaches family members behavioral techniques they can use to modify problematic behaviors evidenced by the dementia patient. One study, for example, found such an approach to be successful not only in reducing or eliminating behavior problems (such as constant talking) but also in increasing the frequency of positive behaviors (such as social behaviors). Recently there have also been efforts to increase the availability of structured day programs for dementia patients, which provide stimulation and social involvement for the patients as well as respite for the family caregivers. The Alzheimer's Association (formerly the Alzheimer's Disease and Related Disorders Association) has support groups throughout the country for families of dementia patients in which information, encouragement, and practical advice on how to manage the patient are offered. The Alzheimer's Association also promotes research, education, and social services for people with dementia and their families.

The Outcome of Cognitive Problems

As discussed earlier, prompt treatment of delirium and reversible dementias usually results in a significant improvement in the condition of the individual. One of the primary goals of a good diagnostic work-up for cognitive difficulties is, in fact, to identify conditions that are remediable or partially remediable. Unfortunately, most individuals with clinically significant cognitive difficulties have progressive conditions that cannot be cured but must simply be managed.

The course of Alzheimer's disease, multi-infarct dementia, and other progressive dementias has not been extensively studied.

There is considerable individual variability in the progress of these illnesses. Some individuals may show a rapid decline in mental and functional abilities, whereas others may evidence cognitive deficits that remain relatively stable for long periods of time with only eventual loss of other abilities.

Psychiatrist Barry Reisberg has suggested that there may be seven different stages to Alzheimer's disease that can be characterized on the basis of certain patterns of problems. These include: (1) no cognitive decline, (2) very mild cognitive decline, (3) mild cognitive decline, (4) moderate cognitive decline, (5) moderately severe cognitive decline, (6) severe cognitive decline, and (7) very severe cognitive decline. Reisberg suggests that clear-cut cognitive difficulties usually do not become apparent until Stage 3, when the individual increasingly becomes, for example, unable to perform in employment or social situations, has difficulty remembering names, and may get lost in unfamiliar locations. By Stage 5 the individual cannot function without the assistance of others. He or she may begin to have difficulty with dressing and may occasionally forget the names of some close family members, as well as experiencing related problems. At Stage 6 the older patient is often unaware of his or her surroundings, the year, or the season; evidences personality changes and emotional disturbances; and may occasionally forget the name of his or her spouse. In the final stage of dementia, the individual has lost virtually all abilities and may be unable to communicate at all, may need help to eat and go to the toilet, and may be unable to walk, among similar deficits. Some mental health researchers have argued that this "staging" of Alzheimer's disease is premature given our still restricted understanding of dementia. Others have found Reisberg's scheme a useful tool for understanding Alzheimer's disease.

The life expectancy of people with Alzheimer's disease, multi-infarct dementia, or other dementias has been subject to widely varying estimates. Mental health professionals have reported that the complete process may last from 2 to 20 years. In part it is difficult to make an estimate of the duration of the illness since early on in the dementing process cognitive symptoms may be so subtle that they are not apparent. Sometimes estimates of the length of the illness are made from the point at which a diagnosis is made. At what point an individual obtains a diagnostic work-up for dementia, however, varies considerably. Some persons, for example, have rather advanced symptoms of dementia before they are formally diagnosed. Nevertheless, estimates of time from the onset of illness to death range from 5 to 8 years and from diagnosis to death, from 3 to 4 years. Most evidence supports the idea that there is greater mortality among persons with dementia than among those without the illness. That is, the life expectancy of persons with dementia is shortened. It is not entirely clear, however, whether dementing illness itself shortens life or whether the increased mortality associated with it results from decreased self-care, susceptibility to pneumonia, poor nutrition, or associated factors. Some researchers have found that people with Alzheimer's disease live longer than people with multi-infarct dementia.

Chapter 3

Other Mental Health Problems

BASIC FACTS

Schizophrenia and Delusional Disorder

- These disorders involve the presence of psychotic symptoms —serious impairments in the individual's ability to accurately perceive reality.

- There are three major types of psychotic symptoms: delusions (false beliefs), hallucinations (false sensory perceptions), and thought disorder (disturbances in the way the individual's thought processes are organized).

- Schizophrenia is a disorder characterized by episodes in which the individual evidences one or several psychotic symptoms.

- Many people with schizophrenia have several episodes and, because of the illness, have difficulties with maintaining normal functioning in the world.

- The onset of schizophrenia is usually early in life.

- There is controversy over whether schizophrenia can appear for the first time in later life.

- The most prominent feature of delusional disorder is the presence of a delusion, the focus of which is often persecutory in nature.

- In contrast to people with schizophrenia, most people with delusional disorders may function adequately on a day-to-day basis.

- The cause of schizophrenia is not known, although research is focusing on genetic factors and defects in brain structure or brain chemistry.

- The cause of delusional disorder has not been well studied but it has been determined that impaired hearing ability is a risk factor for delusional disorder in older adults.

- About 1% of the general population has schizophrenia. The prevalence of the disorder may be the same in younger and older persons. The frequency of delusional disorder among older adults is unknown.

- Treatment of schizophrenia primarily involves administration of anti-psychotic drugs called neuroleptics.

- There is controversy about the best treatment for delusional disorder.

- Treatments do not cure schizophrenia but help to reduce the frequency of psychotic episodes and the severity of symptoms.

Anxiety Disorders

- Although anxiety is a common experience, it may be considered a problem when it interferes with an individual's ability to conduct daily activities and reduces the capacity to experience pleasure.

- Symptoms of anxiety appear to be fairly common among older adults, and, in fact, the elderly are frequent users of anti-anxiety medications. Little research, however, has investigated anxiety disorders among the aged.

- Panic disorder is a condition in which an individual has episodes of extreme fear and discomfort that usually last a few minutes.

- Some symptoms of panic disorder include shortness of breath, dizziness or faintness, sweating, choking, fear of dying, and fear of going crazy.

- Agoraphobia, a condition that often accompanies panic disorder, involves fearfulness about being in a situation from which one might not easily escape if a panic episode occurred.

- As a result of agoraphobia people may avoid crowds, certain forms of transportation, or even going outside unaccompanied.

- Social phobia is an ongoing fear of being scrutinized, embarrassed, or humiliated by others while performing a particular task.

- Social phobias include fear of speaking in public, fear of eating, fear of using public restrooms, or fear that what is said in social situations may not be well received.

- Simple phobia is an ongoing fear of very specific objects or situations.

- Common simple phobias are fear of certain animals, fear of heights, fear of closed spaces, fear of blood, and fear of air travel.

- Obsessive-compulsive disorder is a condition in which the individual has recurring obsessions or compulsions that are severe enough to interfere with emotional, interpersonal, or occupational functioning.

- Obsessions are images, thoughts, or ideas that persistently return.

- Compulsions are actions that are typically performed in response to an obsessional idea.

- Generalized anxiety disorder describes persons who are prone to excessive worrying and anxiety.

- There are a variety of psychological, biological, and environmental theories of the causes of anxiety disorders.

- Treatment of anxiety disorders depends on the type of disorder, although anti-anxiety and other types of psychiatric medications and psychological treatments are often used.

- Most anxiety disorders in younger individuals improve with treatment. Although there is very little research on the treatment of anxiety disorders in older adults, they also appear to benefit by treatment.

Substance Use Disorders

- Although there are a variety of drugs the use of which may become problematic for the individual, alcohol and a class of medication—called sedative, hypnotic, and anxiolytic drugs—are of most concern to older adults.

- Psychoactive substance dependence is the diagnostic term that refers to the most serious form of alcohol or drug problem.

- An individual with psychoactive substance dependence may evidence several of the following problems: The substance is taken over long periods of time, attempts to reduce or control use of the substance are unsuccessful, the substance or substances interfere with the individual's life circumstances, increasingly larger amounts of the substance are needed to achieve the same effect, and withdrawal symptoms may develop when use of the substance is stopped or reduced.

- Psychoactive substance abuse is the use of a substance or substances that causes any of a variety of social, psychological, occupational, or health problems, but these difficulties are neither as severe nor as pervasive as in psychoactive substance dependence.

- Although about 6% of older adults engage in "heavy drinking" probably only 1–2% meet criteria for substance abuse or dependence.

- For two-thirds of older adults with alcohol problems, the difficulties started earlier in life.

- Most studies have found that drug abuse and dependence are almost nonexistent among older adults. This stands in stark contrast to research that indicates that older adults are heavy users of sedatives, hypnotics, or anxiolytics.

- There are a variety of social, psychological, and biological theories about why individuals develop substance use problems.

- Treatment for substance use problems may initially require hospitalization to detoxify the individual. The longer-term goal of treatment is to help the individual abstain from substance use and to help him or her develop better personal and social resources to cope with daily life.

- It appears that most people benefit from alcohol rehabilitation programs. Older persons with later-onset alcoholism appear to do better in treatment than those with lifelong alcohol problems.

- No studies have evaluated the usefulness of treatment for sedative, hypnotic, or anxiolytic abuse or dependence in the aged. Most older adults are, however, likely to benefit from treatment.

Introduction

Although mood and cognitive disorders are the most common difficulties experienced by older adults, there are other mental health problems with which some older people must contend. In fact, *DSM-III-R* lists 17 major classifications of mental disorders that include a total of 208 separate disorders, most of which are potentially applicable to older adults. Although it is not within the scope of this book to fully discuss the range of possible mental health problems of later life, a select group of other difficulties that may appear in or persist into late life will be reviewed in this chapter. These problems include schizophrenia and delusional disorder, anxiety disorders, and substance use disorders. These disorders combined with mood disorders and cognitive disorders constitute the majority of problems evaluated and treated by geriatric mental health practitioners.

As in the previous two chapters, we will address basic questions about these mental health problems.

What are additional mental health problems sometimes experienced by people in later life?

What causes these problems?

How are the problems diagnosed by a mental health professional?

How common are these other mental health problems?

How are these various problems treated?

How effective are the treatments?

Schizophrenia and Delusional Disorder

As was noted in Chapters 1 and 2, mood disorders and cognitive disorders may be accompanied by psychotic symptoms. The term *psychotic* refers to serious impairment in the ability to accurately perceive reality. With mood and cognitive disorders, psychotic symptoms are regarded as associated or secondary features of the illness. That is, they are not the central characteristics of the problem. While a seriously depressed person may, for example, falsely believe, "I am filled with cancer that is eating me alive from the inside out," this belief arises in the context of an emotional disturbance that has secondarily impaired the person's capacity to perceive reality. With schizophrenia and delusional disorder, one or several psychotic symptoms are the central feature of the problem.

There are three major types of psychotic symptoms: delusions, hallucinations, and thought disorder (also known as conceptual disorganization). Delusions are beliefs held by an individual and believed to be true despite clear evidence to the contrary. (An exception is beliefs also held collectively by the individual's culture or subculture that may not be regarded by others as "true," for example, voodoo.) Hallucinations are false sensory perceptions that typically involve hearing things that others do not hear (i.e., auditory hallucinations). Individuals may also see things (visual hallucinations), feel things (somatic or tactile hallucinations), smell things (olfactory hallucinations), or taste things (gustatory hallucinations) that objectively do not exist. Thought disorder refers to disturbances in the way a person's thought processes are organized. For example, an affected individual's thinking may appear fragmented because logical associations between ideas disappear.

Definition

Schizophrenia is a disorder characterized by a variety of psychotic and nonpsychotic symptoms, the onset of which is almost always in early life (for men, typically in the teens and twenties, and for women, usually in the twenties and early thirties). Despite the popular misconception, schizophrenia is *not* "split personality." Multiple personality disorder is, in fact, a different problem entirely, and it is also very rare. For most persons, schizophrenia is a chronic illness in which the individual has an active phase, or episode, during which psychotic symptoms are present. The active phase may be preceded by a period of time (the prodromal phase) in which the person's ability to function on a day-to-day basis is diminished and less dramatic symptoms may be present (for example, strange ideas or behavior). After the active phase of illness ends, the individual enters what is called the residual phase, which may be similar to the prodromal phase. After an active phase, some individuals with schizophrenia do not return to their previous level of functioning. Unfortunately, as time passes, the individual will probably have additional psychotic episodes. The majority of people with schizophrenia will increasingly have difficulties maintaining normal functioning in the outside world, including problems associated with their ability to relate to family, friends, and the work setting. Some mental health professionals have characterized schizophrenia as a chronic, deteriorating illness in which the individual progressively loses a range of previously acquired social, intellectual, emotional, and other resources. There are persons, however, for whom schizophrenia does not have such progressive, devastating effects. Most persons diagnosed with schizophrenia will be required to take medications for this condition for most of their lives. These medications reduce the frequency of episodes of psychotic symptoms but also have a range of side effects that, in themselves, may be problematic.

While the full criteria from *The Diagnostic and Statistical Manual of Mental Disorders (DSM-III-R)* for diagnosing this disorder and others that are reviewed in this book may be found in Appendix B, the following is a summary of the criteria for schizophrenia.

1. One of the following (A, B, or C) must be present in the active phase for at least a week:

A. Two of the following must exist:

Delusions.

Prominent hallucinations (in contrast to symptoms that might be brief or transitory).

Speech that is difficult to understand (incoherence) or speech in which ideas are not clearly or logically related to one another (loosening of association).

Catatonic behavior. This includes a variety of psychomotor behaviors that range from high levels of physical activity to odd posturing of the body (for example, standing on one leg for long periods of time).

The virtual absence of emotional expressiveness (called flat affect) or emotional reactions that do not logically relate to the topic being discussed (inappropriate affect)—for example, laughing while discussing a serious topic.

B. Delusions that are "bizarre" in nature. Bizarre delusions are false beliefs that are wholly unbelievable. For example, an individual may believe that he emits rays from his head that guide airplanes.

C. Prominent hallucinations that involve a voice saying things that are unrelated to depressed or elated emotional states or a voice that maintains an ongoing commentary on things the individual is doing or thinking; or two or more voices that are heard speaking with each other.

2. During the period of difficulty the ability to function (for example, at work and in social relationships) is significantly below the level that existed prior to current difficulties.

3. Other psychiatric disorders (schizoaffective disorder and mood disorders that have psychotic features) must have been discounted as the cause of current difficulties.

4. There must be signs of psychiatric difficulties for at least six months. During this period there must have been an active phase (in which there were psychotic symptoms as described in 1) either with or without the prodromal or residual phases (as described above). (More detailed descriptions of prodromal and residual phase symptoms are offered in the full *DSM-III-R* criteria.)

5. An organic (or neuromedical) factor is not causing difficulties.

6. Certain restrictions exist on assigning a diagnosis of schizophrenia if the individual was previously diagnosed with autism, a psychiatric disorder from infancy or childhood characterized by significant impairment of interpersonal, verbal, and other skills.

Schizophrenia is further classified as to the course of illness (e.g., to what degree it has been chronic or appeared after the age of 45) and characteristic features (i.e., catatonic, disorganized, paranoid, undifferentiated, or residual).

Another disorder in which psychotic symptoms are the central difficulty is delusional disorder. The most prominent feature of this problem is the persistent presence of a delusion, the focus of which is often persecutory in nature. Delusions may also involve sexual or romantic concerns (erotomanic delusions), overestimation of oneself (grandiose delusions), jealousy (jealous delusions), or bodily integrity (somatic delusions). In contrast to schizophrenia, people with delusional disorders may function socially and occupationally in an adequate manner and do not evidence the deteriorating course often seen in schizophrenia.

The following is an outline of *DSM-III-R* diagnostic criteria for delusional disorder.

1. The presence of "nonbizarre" delusions (that is, delusions regarding things that could actually happen in real life).

2. If auditory or visual hallucinations exist, they are not prominent; that is, they are not dominant and persisting features of the current difficulties.

3. The individual does not act oddly or bizarrely apart from the delusion(s).

4. If the individual is experiencing a major depressive episode or a manic syndrome, the duration of this affective episode has been brief relative to the total period of time during which the delusional symptoms have been present.

5. The individual has never met criterion 1 for schizophrenia and the difficulties are not related to organic factors.

A delusional disorder is further classified according to the type of delusion that is present (i.e., erotomanic, grandiose, jealous, persecutory, somatic, or unspecified).

The following are two examples of persons with delusional disorder.

Mary Johnson had reluctantly agreed to be hospitalized. "After all," she said to a psychologist at the time of her hospitalization, "the problem started because of people like you." Ms. Johnson, a 75-year-old, never-married woman who was socially reclusive most of her life, complained of general emotional distress, symptoms of constipation, "ill-formed stools," and a general feeling of weakness. She denied, however, having any symptoms consistent with major mood disorders or hallucinations and showed no evidence of cognitive impairment or significant medical problems. Her difficulties, she contended, had been brought on by medical doctors who, during a recent minor surgical procedure, "punished me for complaints I had previously made to the hospital administration by placing obstructions in my rectum and reducing the flow of blood in my body." She confessed that she had considered suicide one day and had even thought of a method—slashing her wrists. "But then I realized with the reduced blood flow through my veins, I wouldn't have died anyway."

Rose Fortuno was visited by an outreach worker as part of an effort by a local social service agency to visit community elderly to determine if they had social service or psychiatric needs for which services could be arranged. Mrs. Fortuno, a pleasant elderly woman who described herself as an "undiscovered writer," said that she had moved into the local neighborhood a few years after a divorce from her husband. Mrs. Fortuno said she had a relatively satisfying life that included frequent concert-going, participation in a literary society, and ongoing efforts to get her romance novels published. As the outreach worker was about to leave, Mrs. Fortuno noted that there was one problem with which she needed help, but, she confessed, she was reluctant to discuss it.

"The divorce with my husband was an ugly affair. The worst of it, however, was the aftermath. In retaliation, my husband enlisted the FBI to harass me. At first they simply followed me, but after a while that did not satisfy them. A few months ago, while I was sleeping on the couch in the living room, they drilled holes through the floor and into the couch through which they injected me with mind-altering drugs. Things really got out of hand a few weeks ago. While I was asleep, the FBI entered my apartment and implanted a mechanical device in my right knee that, on radio command, locks my knee. I can cope with things during the week but on weekends I become especially fearful. Do you think it is possible to arrange to have someone stay with me on weekends?"

The outreach worker empathized with how fearful these things must be and said that he knew a social worker who might be able to help. An appointment was arranged with a psychiatric social worker. When, at this meeting, Mrs. Fortuno learned that the social worker was employed at a community mental health center, she politely declined further services from the social worker.

A few months later the outreach worker saw Mrs. Fortuno limping down one of the neighborhood streets. When she saw the outreach worker she smiled and greeted him warmly. She pointed to her right knee and

remarked, "See! I told you they could lock my knee."
Although she said she appreciated the outreach worker's
efforts to help her, she did not believe her problem
required psychiatric assistance.

Despite the fact that schizophrenia is an illness with onset in
early life, it concerns older adults for two reasons. First, there are
older adults who have suffered from schizophrenia since early
life and continue to suffer from it. Many of these individuals
were placed in state psychiatric institutions early in life, and
some of them were later "discharged to the community" during
the reduction of the populations of state psychiatric hospitals in
the 1960s and 1970s. Many of those residing "in the community"
actually live in nursing homes that have taken the place of state
hospitals in many areas of the country. Second, a very small
number of older adults may evidence the first signs of schizophrenia or psychotic symptomatology similar to schizophrenia
in later life. There is, however, considerable controversy regarding this second issue.

Until the latest revision of *DSM-III-R,* it was believed that
schizophrenia could not be diagnosed after the age of 45. The
reasoning was, in part, that since schizophrenia characteristically
appeared very early in life it was unlikely that the onset of even
very similar symptoms in senescence was the same disorder. This
position was particularly popular in the United States. Some
schools of European psychiatry took a different point of view
and essentially argued that schizophrenia was schizophrenia no
matter when the age of onset. As part of his larger studies of
late-life mental disorders, the British psychiatrist Sir Martin
Roth, who was discussed in earlier chapters, suggested that
schizophrenia-like symptoms with onset late in life should be
called late paraphrenia. The term *paraphrenia* was borrowed
from a term (then in disuse) that had been coined by the German
psychiatrist Emil Kraepelin. Kraepelin had used *paraphrenia* to
describe a form of psychotic illness characterized by paranoid
delusions and an absence of some of the cognitive and affective
difficulties seen in schizophrenia. He believed this pattern of
symptoms was different from schizophrenia. Given that late-
onset psychoses are often dominated by paranoid delusions in
persons with relatively intact personalities, this term appeared to

Sir Martin Roth to best describe this phenomenon. Some gero-psychiatrists continue to favor this description.

The current consensus is, however, that schizophrenia can appear in late life and that its symptoms can be differentiated from those of a delusional disorder and other disorders. Further research will determine whether late-onset schizophrenia-like illness is indeed part of a disorder that typically begins in early life or is a different form of mental illness.

Frequency

As should be apparent from the above discussion, documenting the frequency of schizophrenia and delusional disorder is difficult since, over the years, mental health professionals have used different definitions to describe them. Some research, however, allows us to draw a few conclusions. It appears that less than 1 percent of older adults (usually defined as 65 years or older) have schizophrenia. (About 1 percent of the general population have schizophrenia.) At least 90 percent of older adults with schizophrenia experienced the onset of the disorder in earlier life. The frequency of delusional disorder among older adults is not known. In one recent study in the United States, almost 8 percent of older adults evidenced one symptom of schizophrenia, 4.3 percent showed significant delusional symptoms, and 5.4 percent showed significant symptoms of hallucination. Of course, the cause or causes of these symptoms could be attributed to any number of different factors.

Possible Causes

The cause of schizophrenia is not known. Current theories suggest there may be a general genetic vulnerability to schizophrenia that, when combined with other factors, will trigger the illness.

Schizophrenia is more common in some families. Each child of a person with schizophrenia, for example, has a 10 percent chance of developing schizophrenia. Studies have found that the likelihood of both of a pair of identical twins having schizophrenia is higher than that for fraternal twins. Other research has found that even children of schizophrenic parents who were adopted and raised by other parents are at greater risk for schizophrenia than others.

Recent research has suggested that one important component of schizophrenia may be defects in brain chemistry, particularly in neurotransmitters (chemical substances involved in the transmission of information within the brain). Other research has investigated the possibility that structural abnormalities in the brain are related to schizophrenia. The development of the CT scan (computerized axial tomography, a diagnostic device that takes multiple X-rays of the brain), the PET scan (positron emission tomography, an instrument that measures the metabolic activity of the brain), and the MRI scan (magnetic resonance imaging, a machine that can precisely measure structures in the brain using a magnetic field) offers new opportunities to more carefully examine brain changes associated with schizophrenia and other illnesses. Although some differences in brain structure and metabolism between people with schizophrenia and people without it have been identified in research using these instruments, findings are at present regarded as tentative.

In previous years some mental health professionals speculated that the cause of schizophrenia lay in certain patterns of child rearing. This is now regarded as unlikely. Most current efforts are devoted to helping parents of people with schizophrenia to learn how to better cope with the practical and emotional difficulties that arise from having a family member with this disorder.

The cause of delusional disorder has not been well studied. Factors thought to be associated with its late-life onset have been grouped with late-life schizophrenia (that is, both disorders have been called late-life paraphrenia). Late-life onset psychotic illness is thought to have a genetic component, although to a lesser degree than that found in schizophrenia of early onset. One theory is that some people have a form of schizophrenia that, for unknown reasons, does not express itself until late life. Sensory impairment, most notably deafness, has been associated with increased risk for psychotic symptoms, particularly symptoms of paranoia. Some have suggested that deafness can "elicit" schizophrenia in a person who otherwise would not have experienced it. Others have postulated that sensory deprivation may incline the individual to construct idiosyncratic ideas that slowly become organized into delusions. People with lifelong personality disorders, people who evidence behavior regarded as eccentric or reclusive, or people who relate poorly to other people have also been thought to be predisposed to later-life psychotic illness.

Evaluation

General principles for a thorough diagnostic evaluation of an older person with psychiatric difficulties have been outlined in Chapters 1 and 2. These include establishing a good rapport with the older individual and family members, taking a thorough recent and past history of difficulties, considering a wide range of other organic and nonorganic possible causes of current difficulties, and making sure that the older adult's medical condition and current medications have been evaluated. Evaluating the presence of sensory deficits (e.g., visual and auditory problems) is important because such deficits are associated with delusional symptoms. Since psychotic symptoms may be part of other disorders, it is imperative that they be considered. The possibility that, for example, psychotic symptoms are part of a mood disorder that is accompanied by delusions (e.g., major depression or bipolar disorder), a delirium, or dementia is particularly critical to consider. Given the rarity of late-onset schizophrenia, in fact, the presence of psychotic symptoms is more likely to signal the presence of one of these problems than of schizophrenia. On the other hand, given the infrequency of late-onset psychotic disorders, schizophrenia could be easily overlooked when, in fact, it exists.

Treatment

Treatment of schizophrenia primarily involves administration of anti-psychotic drugs called neuroleptics (also known as major tranquilizers). In the 1950s the neuroleptic chlorpromazine began to be used in the United States. It was a revolution for psychiatry since neuroleptics were the first truly effective treatment for controlling a variety of psychotic symptoms including delusions, hallucinations, thought disorder (conceptual disorganization), and aggressive and disorganized behavior. The introduction of neuroleptics allowed many people with schizophrenia to live outside of state psychiatric institutions. Like many medications, however, neuroleptics have side effects against which the therapeutic advantages of the drug must be weighed.

Neuroleptic drugs are thought to alter the brain neurotransmitter dopamine, which is believed to play a critical role in the expression of psychiatric symptoms. There are a variety of neuroleptic medications that are all regarded as generally effective. Usually the choice of a neuroleptic will depend on its characteristic side effects. Neuroleptics are sometimes classified according to their potency (i.e., low potency, intermediate potency, and high potency). Higher amounts of low-potency drugs are required to achieve the same effect as lower doses of high-potency drugs. Examples of neuroleptics of different potencies include:

1. Low potency: chlorpromazine (trade name Thorazine) and thioridazine (trade name Mellaril)

2. Intermediate potency: perphenazine (Trilafon), loxapine succinate (Loxitane), and molindone HC1 (Moban)

3. High potency: haloperidol (Haldol), thiothixene (Navane), fluphenazine HC1 (Prolixin), and trifluoperazine HC1 (Stelazine)

Most of these medications are prescribed by tablet or, occasionally, are administered in liquid form. A few are administered intramuscularly (that is, by injection) and need only be given intermittently. An alphabetical list of trade names of common neuroleptics and other psychotropic medications may be found in Appendix A.

Adults with schizophrenia who are now in their sixties are the first cohort of aged who have had the benefit of neuroleptic medications throughout most of their lives. As noted, many such persons with schizophrenia were discharged from large state psychiatric institutions in the 1960s and 1970s and currently reside in nursing homes. Very little has been written about the social and psychiatric condition of these individuals or about what might be optimal psychiatric or psychosocial treatments for them. For people with schizophrenia, prescription of neuroleptics should be based on the kind of symptoms that are evident, the medical condition of the individual, the possible side effects from neuroleptics, and the therapeutic effectiveness of the medication.

As discussed in some detail in Chapter 1, the manner in which older people metabolize drugs in their bodies differs somewhat from that of younger individuals. The primary purpose of psychotropic drugs, as with neuroleptics, is to change brain chemistry.

The means by which the medications make their way to the brain depend on how the drug gets into the system (absorption), how it is dispersed throughout the system (distribution), and how the drug is eventually eliminated from the system (elimination). Neuroleptics are absorbed somewhat more slowly and distributed and eliminated less efficiently as people age. As a result it takes longer for neuroleptics to reach levels within the system that are therapeutic (that is, enough of the drug is in the system to have the intended effect), and it also takes longer for the older person to eliminate the medication from his or her system. The practical implication of these factors is that older people usually need smaller doses of neuroleptics, tend to be more sensitive to the side effects of the drugs, and take longer to eliminate the medications from their systems.

There are a number of possible side effects from neuroleptics. These include orthostatic hypotension, sedation, and anticholinergic and extrapyramidal side effects. Low-potency neuroleptics are usually associated with sedation, orthostatic hypotension, and anticholinergic side effects. High-potency neuroleptics are more likely to result in extrapyramidal side effects. These side effects are discussed below.

As reviewed in Chapter 1, orthostatic hypotension is a sudden drop of blood pressure that occurs particularly when an individual sits up or stands up quickly. The most immediate danger is that the person will fall. With older people this may result in bone fracture. Sedation, of course, is best characterized as drowsiness. Anticholinergic side effects are associated with dry mouth, constipation, retention of urine, and other problems. Neuroleptic medications may also less commonly lead to a condition called central nervous system anticholinergic toxicity, which may result in disorientation, confusion, impaired recent memory, and even visual hallucinations and assaultive behavior.

Neuroleptics may also cause extrapyramidal symptoms, including an acute dystonic reaction (spasms of the back, neck, face, and other muscles), akathisia (restlessness, muscular tension, and an urge to constantly be moving), akinesia (lack of energy, reduced motivation, a "blankness," and other problems), and Parkinson-like symptoms (symptoms often seen in Parkinson's disease such as drooling and a shuffling walk). Extrapyramidal side effects are usually treated by reducing the amount of

medication or prescribing anticholinergic drugs such as diphenhydramine hydrochloride (trade name Benadryl) or benztropine
mesylate (Cogentin).

Tardive dyskinesia (TD) is a side effect of neuroleptics that
may be irreversible. It is characterized by a range of involuntary
muscle movements including facial grimacing, lip smacking, jaw
movements, tics, and tongue movements. People with the most
severe cases of TD may have difficulty speaking, walking, eating,
or even breathing, although these symptoms are quite rare. Usually the symptoms of TD come on gradually. Older people are
more susceptible to developing TD, however, and symptoms
may become evident even after relatively brief exposure to neuroleptic medications. Some estimates are that 40 percent of people over the age of 60 who are treated with neuroleptics will
develop TD. Symptoms of TD may improve or disappear after
neuroleptics are stopped, although this is less likely in older
people than in younger individuals.

Obviously neuroleptics are powerful medications—powerful
enough to dampen or eliminate severe psychiatric symptoms as
well as to induce a wide range of side effects, some of which are
irreversible. Psychiatrists must carefully weigh the benefits and
risks of these medications. Unfortunately, neuroleptics are sometimes inappropriately prescribed to older persons, particularly
by community physicians.

Martin McHugh was evaluated at the geriatric mental
health clinic for a second opinion about the medication
he had been receiving for several years from his family
physician for "anxiety." When evaluated, he had no
apparent psychiatric symptoms. What was most notable
was his persistent lip-smacking, tongue movements, and
facial grimacing, about which Mr. McHugh made no
comment. He seemed unfamiliar with the medication he
had been taking for "anxiety."

With information gained from other family members,
the following scenario emerged. Shortly after retirement,
Mr. McHugh experienced feelings of anxiety and
depression, for which his physician prescribed a
neuroleptic—a medication that should not have been
prescribed for the problems that were described.

Mr. McHugh continued to take the medication despite the fact that he no longer experienced feelings of anxiety and depression. The involuntary muscle movements observed were apparently tardive dyskinesia. The neuroleptic medication was discontinued, but, unfortunately, the symptoms of tardive dyskinesia did not diminish. It appeared that Mr. McHugh would be left with permanent side effects from a medication that should not have been prescribed in the first place.

When neuroleptics are prescribed for an older adult, side effects must be carefully evaluated. Since discontinuation of neuroleptics at the first sign of TD makes it more likely that the condition will not be permanent, vigilance by the psychiatrist regarding TD-related problems is important. In general, people with schizophrenia are treated indefinitely with neuroleptics. Sometimes psychiatrists stop neuroleptics for limited periods of time called drug holidays and later restart the medication. The medical condition of some older people and side effects acquired from neuroleptics, however, may require stopping the medication altogether.

There is some controversy about the best treatment for delusional disorder. Some psychiatrists have reported that neuroleptics do not significantly diminish delusions and therefore argue against their use. Other mental health professionals feel that the older patient with delusional disorder should be prescribed a neuroleptic for a period of time to ascertain whether the medication will be useful. Given the possible side effects associated with neuroleptics, if this medication is prescribed, it should be given for no longer than the time required to determine its utility for the patient. Some mental health professionals have found that older persons with delusions who are living alone and have no significant social contact improve without medication when more frequent interactions with other people are made available.

Mental health professionals working with people with schizophrenia or delusional disorder must slowly and sensitively establish a trusting and supportive relationship with the older individual. This is accomplished in part by not initially challenging the veracity of the older person's symptoms, but rather empathizing with the emotional distress that he or she must be feeling because of those symptoms. Close coordination with the families or significant others of older people with these problems is important for the monitoring of symptoms and intelligent treatment planning. Some older people with these disorders may benefit by supportive individual or group psychotherapy during which they may discuss past and current difficulties.

Older adults with these disorders may periodically have to be hospitalized. This is particularly true for those suffering from schizophrenia who, during the active phase of illness, may become so disorganized by psychotic symptoms that they cannot function independently. For most, once symptoms of psychosis have subsided, return to prior living arrangements is possible.

Effectiveness of Treatments

Current treatments for schizophrenia do not cure the disorder but simply help to manage it. Neuroleptic medications have been shown to have a significant effect on controlling the frequency of episodes of psychosis (the active phase). Studies of younger persons with schizophrenia have found that, after a psychotic episode, only 40 percent of those who remained on medication relapsed within two years, while 80 percent of those not on medication relapsed in two years. There is some evidence to suggest that neuroleptics are at least as effective in older persons as in younger individuals with schizophrenia.

Overall, the prognosis for people with the onset of schizophrenia in early life is not particularly good. Even with treatment most will continue to have episodes in which they experience symptoms of psychosis and will live under reduced social and economic circumstances. Some have observed, however, that among older people with early-onset schizophrenia symptoms become less severe in old age. The prognosis for late-onset schizophrenia and probably for delusional disorder (again, both have usually been called late paraphrenia) is better. Some mental health professionals have found that people with late-onset psychotic illness seem to respond better to neuroleptic medications than do older people with early-onset schizophrenia. There is virtually no research on the usefulness of psychological or supportive services for older people with either early- or late-onset psychoses.

Anxiety Disorders

Of all the disorders included in *DSM-III-R* almost one-quarter involve symptoms of anxiety. Among anxiety disorders, there are nine separate classifications. Anxiety problems appear to be one of the most common mental health difficulties of older adults, and older people tend to be frequent users of anti-anxiety medications. Despite this, there is very little research on anxiety disorders in older people.

In view of the large number of anxiety disorders classified by *DSM-III-R* and the paucity of research about such disorders in the aged, I will provide only an overview of some issues on this topic. This will include a discussion of generalized anxiety disorder, panic disorders, phobias, and obsessive-compulsive disorder. Although the *DSM-III-R* criteria will not be summarized in the text, the complete criteria for these disorders are available in Appendix B.

Definition

Anxiety is a common experience for most people. There are a wide variety of circumstances in life that should reasonably elicit anxiety. Late-life changes such as physical illness, loss of friends and relatives, changed economic circumstances, and altered social roles all make older adults more vulnerable to anxiety. Anxiety may be considered a problem when it interferes with an individual's ability to conduct daily activities and reduces the capacity to experience pleasure. Nevertheless, there is controversy regarding at what point anxiety crosses the line from being a normal response to life circumstances and becomes a disorder. In addition, symptoms of anxiety accompany many mental health problems and there is not complete consensus among mental health professionals about which difficulties should be classified as anxiety disorders rather than as some other disorders.

Panic disorder is a condition in which an individual has episodes of extreme fear and discomfort that usually last a few minutes and that, at the outset of the disorder, come on unexpectedly. As the condition progresses, however, certain situations may trigger a panic episode. An individual may experience several symptoms, some of which include shortness of breath, dizziness or faintness, sweating, choking, fear of dying, and fear of going crazy. Many persons with the condition subsequently develop an associated problem known as agoraphobia. Agoraphobia is fearfulness about being in a situation from which one might not be able to easily escape if a panic episode occurred. For example, people with agoraphobia may avoid crowds, certain forms of transportation, or even going outside unaccompanied. Panic disorder is therefore diagnosed as with or without agoraphobia. Some individuals, however, may have agoraphobia as the primary difficulty and not have accompanying panic attacks. This is considered a separate disorder that is known as agoraphobia without history of panic disorder. This condition is rarely seen by mental health professionals among people seeking treatment although it exists in the population at large.

Grace Carlisle reluctantly agreed to answer the door when the social service outreach worker knocked. She finally allowed him to enter after considerable negotiating. Mrs. Carlisle, who was dressed in a shabby housecoat, lived in a dimly lit apartment in which the window shades were pulled down. She said she was embarrassed about her appearance but that she had not been able to shop in recent years.

Mrs. Carlisle said that she had been subject to "spells" ever since she was a young woman in which she felt nauseated, dizzy, shaky, short of breath, and "felt like I was going crazy." As a result, she had avoided going out for fear of the embarrassment she would feel if other people saw her having such a "spell." She said that over the years her husband had been sympathetic about her condition and never pushed her to leave the home very often. After her husband died, however, life became increasingly difficult. Since she and her husband did not have children and Mrs. Carlisle had virtually no friends, it was necessary for her to venture out of her home more frequently than ever before. On a brief trip to the local grocery market five years before she had been attacked by a man who stole her purse. After that she never left her apartment, having arranged for the superintendent of her building to buy her groceries once a week.

At one point in the conversation Mrs. Carlisle opened one of the window shades, looked outside, and said, "It's spring, isn't it? My, would I like to make one more trip back to the little farm where I was born in New Hampshire. I am getting on in years, you know." The outreach worker said he would see what could be done so that Mrs. Carlisle might be better able to make a trip to see her birthplace.

Subsequently, a psychiatrist visited Mrs. Carlisle in her home, diagnosed a panic disorder with agoraphobia, and prescribed medication. A psychiatric social worker met with Mrs. Carlisle on a weekly basis to assist her in better arranging her affairs. This included a visit to a physician, who identified a variety of medical problems that needed attention.

A few months later the psychiatric social worker telephoned the outreach worker and said that Mrs. Carlisle was eagerly planning a trip to take a final look at the New Hampshire farm on which she had been raised.

Social phobia is an ongoing fear of being scrutinized, embarrassed, or humiliated by others while performing a particular task. A common social phobia is fear of speaking in public. Others include fear of eating, fear of using public restrooms, or fear that what is said in social situations may not be well received. As a consequence, individuals will avoid these situations or engage in them with considerable anxiety. Of course, some degree of anxiety is experienced by most people in certain public or social situations, but the extent and consequences of social phobias are what make them disorders.

Simple phobia is an ongoing fear of very specific objects or situations. The most common phobias are fear of certain animals (e.g., dogs, mice, insects, or snakes) but also include fear of heights, closed spaces, blood, and air travel. When confronted with the object of phobia the individual will have anxiety-related symptoms such as sweating, heart pounding, and problems with breathing. People with simple phobias may avoid situations in which they might be confronted with the object of the phobia, and, as a result, the condition may seriously interfere with the person's ability to carry on usual activities.

Obsessive-compulsive disorder is a condition in which the individual has recurring obsessions or compulsions that are severe enough to interfere with emotional, interpersonal, or occupational functioning. Obsessions are images, thoughts, or ideas that persistently return and that, at least in the beginning, are regarded by the individual as senseless. A common obsession is thoughts about violence (for example, a man has thoughts about killing his wife even though he loves her). The individual usually tries to stop the obsessional thoughts in one manner or another. Compulsions are actions that are typically performed in response to an obsessional idea. Compulsive rituals span a variety of behaviors including cleaning (e.g., very frequent washing of hands), repeating (e.g., saying a word over and over to ward off injury to self or others), checking (e.g., checking repeatedly to be sure that the oven has been turned off), completing (e.g., engaging in a complicated series of steps that must be started again from the beginning if any one of them is completed incorrectly), and hoarding (e.g., saving several years' worth of newspapers). If there is an attempt to resist either the obsession or the compulsion, the individual experiences tension and anxiety that is relieved only if the thought or act is completed.

The social service outreach worker was asked by an area landlord to visit Katherine Gilespie because she was on the verge of being evicted for living in an apartment that was described as a "fire trap."

When the outreach worker entered Ms. Gilespie's apartment, he found it filled with newspapers, toilet paper rolls, and empty tissue boxes stacked in six-foot piles. The apartment was entirely filled with paper with only small spaces in which to walk or sit. Ms. Gilespie said she was indeed a "collector" but that she found the landlord's demand that she remove the large volume of paper from her apartment to be unreasonable. She said she had spent countless hours organizing and reorganizing the paper and the thought of losing it made her very anxious.

Ms. Gilespie was referred to the local community mental health center, where she received treatment for her compulsion. She eventually agreed to have the paper removed from her apartment and consequently was not evicted.

Generalized anxiety disorder describes persons who are prone to excessive worrying and anxiety. It is accompanied by sets of specific symptoms including those associated with motor tension (e.g., restlessness and trembling), autonomic hyperactivity (e.g., shortness of breath, sweating, dry mouth, and nausea), and vigilance and scanning (e.g., feeling tense, problems with concentration, and trouble falling asleep). This condition does not usually impair a person's day-to-day functioning.

> Laura Kelty came to the geriatric mental health clinic complaining of being a "high-strung" person inclined to "fret" about things and to exaggerate the importance of difficulties that confronted her. Mrs. Kelty said that her husband had always been of great help in "keeping things in perspective" and "calming me down." Since his death a few years ago, she felt that her anxiety problems had grown worse. The onset of some minor health problems a year ago had triggered a never-ending series of concerns about her health that she described as "unrealistic." "Every little ache and pain I think is a heart problem or cancer. This is silly, I know. But I don't know how to stop it." The more anxious Mrs. Kelty became, the more likely she would experience physical symptoms of anxiety like heart palpitations and diarrhea, which caused her to further worry whether she had physical health problems.

All of these disorders commonly first appear in early or middle life. It is very rare that a person would experience any of these conditions for the first time in late life.

Frequency

Most research findings on the frequency of anxiety problems among the aged have used *DSM-III* criteria, which are somewhat different from those in *DSM-III-R*. Generalized anxiety disorder appears to be the most common of anxiety disorders (7.1 percent frequency was reported in one study among people aged 65 to 79). In other research studies prevalence rates among people 60 years or older ranged from 1 percent to 5.5 percent for agoraphobia,

0.7 percent to 12.5 percent for simple phobias, and 0.1 percent to 0.4 percent for panic disorders. Women have been found to have higher rates of anxiety disorders than men, and anxiety disorders are less common among older people than in younger individuals.

Many mental health professionals believe that current diagnostic categories do not fully capture the range of anxiety-related problems experienced by older individuals. For example, different individual symptoms of anxiety are fairly common among older people, although the majority of these individuals do not meet *DSM-III-R* criteria for a disorder.

Possible Causes

There are different theories about the origins of anxiety. Early psychoanalytic theorists posited that anxiety was a symptom that signaled the presence of underlying conflicts from childhood (usually related to issues of sex and/or aggression). Psychoanalytic treatment involved an attempt to uncover and resolve the presumed conflict. Learning theory states that anxiety is a behavior that is learned like any other behavior. For example, an individual who is fearful of closed-in spaces "learns" that anxiety can be relieved by avoiding such spaces. Unfortunately, avoidance may severely limit the range of physical environments in which the person can function. Another view of anxiety is biological. Recent research has identified certain biochemical changes associated with anxiety disorders. Whether biochemical changes are the cause or consequence of different anxiety problems (or both) remains to be determined.

Finally, environmental stress may trigger symptoms of anxiety. Late-life problems including physical illness, social role changes, reduced economic resources, and the deaths of friends and family can precipitate anxiety symptoms in older adults. How life stresses may precipitate the onset of anxiety *disorders*, however, is not well understood.

Evaluation

As discussed, a thorough evaluation of current and past mental health difficulties, medical conditions, current medications, social and familial circumstances, and daily activities is important in diagnosing mental health problems. Determining whether anxiety symptoms are medical or psychiatric in origin is one of the more difficult diagnostic problems since anxiety-related symptoms can have physical manifestations (e.g., sweating, heart pounding, or restlessness). To further complicate the issue, people with diagnosed medical problems may become quite anxious in response to those problems.

Treatment

Most anxiety-related problems among both younger and older people are treated with medication, behavioral therapy, or a combination of treatments. Medication is the most common method of treating anxiety problems.

Benzodiazepines are a type of medication most often used in the treatment of generalized anxiety disorder. Benzodiazepines are part of a group of drugs called sedatives, hypnotics, and anxiolytics. Benzodiazepines are also sometimes used in the treatment of panic disorder. Although no type of benzodiazepine has been found to be more effective than any other, these medications differ in the speed with which they are eliminated from the system. As has been discussed, older individuals metabolize drugs differently from younger persons. Older people eliminate benzodiazepines from their systems more slowly than younger individuals and are therefore more vulnerable to possible side effects. Benzodiazepines are usually classified as either short acting or long acting. An example of a short-acting benzodiazepine is lorazepam (Ativan); an example of a long-acting benzodiazepine is diazepam (Valium). Common side effects from benzodiazepines include sedation, fatigue, and drowsiness. Some have also suggested that benzodiazepines may interfere with certain memory processes, although others have found that the medications may improve memory in some individuals. In general, however, most mental health professionals do not feel that benzodiazepines significantly affect memory.

The advantage of short-acting benzodiazepines is that side effects are less likely to occur because the drug is quickly eliminated from the system. The disadvantage of short-acting benzodiazepines is that people must take them two to three times a day. The advantage of long-acting benzodiazepines is that the individual needs to take the medication only once a day or, in the case of older adults, once every two days. The disadvantage of long-acting benzodiazepines is that there is an increased risk that the medication will build up in the system and cause increasing sedation, fatigue, and drowsiness. Benzodiazepines should be prescribed in small doses using the short-acting variety whenever possible. Benzodiazepines are not generally recommended for patients with dementia because these drugs may aggravate the condition. The medications may, however, have a role in managing agitation in some patients.

Other caveats are important in prescribing benzodiazepines. One possible problem is that people sometimes become dependent on this type of medication and have difficulty stopping it. For some, there may be symptoms of withdrawal accompanied by, for example, feelings of apprehension, tremors, agitation, stomach upset, and sweating. Although occasionally it may be necessary to prescribe benzodiazepines for longer periods of time, the potential for dependency on the drug must be weighed against its therapeutic benefit. Another potential side effect of benzodiazepines is that, since this drug sedates the central nervous system, it may cause confusion, memory loss, or associated symptoms when the individual is also taking drugs that depress the central nervous system (e.g., alcohol, narcotics, some antidepressants, and neuroleptics).

Another type of medication occasionally used in the treatment of generalized anxiety disorder is beta-adrenergic blocking agents, or beta-blockers. Beta-blockers are primarily used in the treatment of high blood pressure, certain heart conditions, and migraine headaches. For people with anxiety problems accompanied by severe physical symptoms of anxiety (e.g., tremors, heart pounding, sweating, and muscle tension), this type of medication may be useful. The most well known beta-blocker is propranolol (trade name Inderal). People sometimes take a single dose of propranolol prior to confronting certain social phobias (for example, public speaking). The drug often reduces anxiety enough so that the individual may function more effectively. Propranolol tends to lower blood pressure and therefore people taking the medication must be monitored carefully.

Antidepressant medications are used to treat certain anxiety problems. Some persons being evaluated for mental health problems may primarily complain of anxiety, but closer evaluation reveals that the symptom is part of a major depression. Treatment of the depression with antidepressants will usually reduce anxiety symptoms. Panic disorder is primarily treated with antidepressants. Obsessive-compulsive disorder is also sometimes treated with antidepressants. The drug clomipramine (trade name Anafranil) has been found by some researchers to be effective in reducing obsessive-compulsive symptoms. Other antidepressants (fluvoxamine and fluoxetine) have shown some promise in the treatment of obsessive-compulsive disorder but are currently considered experimental for obsessive-compulsive disorder.

Before the introduction of benzodiazepines in the United States, a type of drugs called barbiturates were used for the treatment of anxiety. Examples of barbiturates include amobarbital (trade name Amytal) and meprobamate (Miltown). These medications are generally considered as outmoded in the treatment of anxiety conditions because they pose a greater risk than benzodiazepines for the development of dependence, side effects, and serious withdrawal symptoms. Antihistamines such as diphenhydramine (Benadryl) are occasionally used in treating anxiety for people with certain health conditions (for example, chronic obstructive lung disease) that benzodiazepines would adversely affect.

Behavioral therapy techniques have proven to be quite useful in the treatment of phobias and obsessive-compulsive disorders. The foundation of behavioral therapy for phobias is repeatedly confronting the object or situation that causes anxiety until the anxiety significantly diminishes or stops. For example, a person who fears cats will be placed in a situation where he or she must spend time with a cat. Although initially the person may feel considerable anxiety, this feeling typically dissipates. There are a variety of ways to conduct behavioral therapy. One method is to expose the individual to the feared object by asking the patient to mentally imagine being in close proximity to it; another is to gradually expose the person to the object of phobia (desensitization). Yet another technique abruptly confronts the individual with the feared object (this is called flooding). Other methods that involve teaching the individual ways to gradually reduce the frequency of problematic behaviors exist to help people with obsessive-compulsive disorder.

As noted earlier, psychoanalytic theory posits that certain anxiety problems reflect the presence of deep underlying conflicts. Coming to terms with the conflict should therefore reduce symptoms of anxiety. Little research supports this approach, however, and most believe that medication and behavior therapy are the best treatments for anxiety disorders. It is important to emphasize, however, that some health professionals are too quick to prescribe medication to treat anxiety symptoms in older people. Identification of the cause or causes of anxiety problems is critical. Helping the older individual who has certain symptoms of anxiety or generalized anxiety disorder to identify environmental, behavioral, or cognitive precipitants of anxiety may help to reduce feelings of anxiety. Sometimes psychotherapy is done in lieu of medication, sometimes it is done in conjunction with medication.

Effectiveness of Treatments

There is almost no research that has evaluated the usefulness of different treatments in the alleviation of anxiety disorders in the aged. In studies with younger individuals, behavioral therapies have been proven successful in treating phobias and obsessive-compulsive disorder when compared with no treatment. Medications have also been found successful in the treatment of generalized anxiety disorder, panic disorder, and obsessive-compulsive disorder when compared with placebos (inactive substances given in pill form that are typically used in research studies). Although these treatments have been judged to be successful, success has been measured by different criteria. For certain phobias and panic disorder, treatment success may be judged as complete disappearance of symptoms. For problems like obsessive-compulsive disorder, reduction in the frequency and severity of problematic behaviors is judged to be a successful outcome. Sometimes several approaches used together have been found more successful than a single approach. Future efforts will seek to create new treatments that are more effective for larger numbers of persons than existing treatments.

Substance Use Disorders

The idea that older adults abuse alcohol and drugs does not fit conventional images of the elderly as stable citizens who set an example for younger generations. Substance abuse is generally portrayed as a young person's problem and, in fact, most substance use problems do exist among younger individuals. Alcohol and drug problems also occur, however, among a select group of older individuals, and diagnosis and treatment of these problems can improve the mental and physical well-being of these older adults.

Alcohol has played a role in social and ceremonial aspects of human life throughout recorded history. Although various cultures hold different attitudes about the use of alcohol, alcohol is often regarded with some ambivalence. The majority of individuals in this society drink alcohol to some extent, and for most it is a pleasurable experience shared with family and friends. For some who drink, alcohol progressively impairs social, occupational, and family functioning.

Other psychoactive (that is, mind-altering) drugs have also been available to people throughout history, but in recent years in this society we have witnessed the widespread availability of legal and illegal psychoactive drugs other than alcohol. These have been the cause of significant personal and social problems. Older adults are not immune to drug-related problems. For example, at a recent professional meeting on overmedication of the elderly, drug use among older adults was referred to as "the nation's *other* drug problem." Some mental health professionals believe medical doctors have overly relied on prescribing drugs to the elderly, especially psychoactive drugs (such as anti-anxiety medications), in lieu of psychological and social treatments. Nevertheless, older adults live in a society in which drug use is widespread and they, like younger individuals, are vulnerable to the difficulties associated with overreliance on such substances.

Definition

Although there are a wide variety of substance use problems, we will focus on those that are of most concern to older adults: (1) alcohol and (2) sedative, hypnotic, and anxiolytic drugs. Alcohol and drugs have a wide range of effects on individuals. Determining when these substances are used in an appropriate social or therapeutic manner versus when they are abused has not always been easy. Criteria outlined in the section in *DSM-III-R* titled "Psychoactive Substance Dependence" reflect conventional thinking about what constitutes significant drug and alcohol problems. The *DSM-III-R* criteria are broad and encompass a variety of problems associated with many different legal and illegal substances.

A general summary of the *DSM-III-R* criteria for psychoactive substance dependence follows.

1. At least three of the following difficulties are evident:

   The substance has been taken over periods of time and in amounts that exceeded what the individual intended.

   There is an ongoing desire for the substance or the person has tried, without success, to reduce or control taking it.

   Considerable time is spent obtaining the substance, taking the substance, and recovering from its effects.

   Intoxication (that is, the effects of the substance on the central nervous system) and withdrawal symptoms frequently interfere with the person's ability to carry on usual activities.

   Important life activities are stopped or curtailed because of substance use.

   Even though the individual knows that use of the substance is causing psychological, social, or health problems, he or she continues.

   Significant tolerance (defined as at least a 50% increase over what was initially used) for the substance develops. Tolerance is the need for larger and larger amounts of the substance in order to achieve the same effect.

Withdrawal symptoms develop that are characteristic of the substance that is being used. Withdrawal symptoms and tolerance are part of a dependency syndrome. Withdrawal symptoms are the physical and mental effects of stopping substance use. For example, some symptoms of alcohol withdrawal include sweating, irritability, headaches, and insomnia.

The individual takes the substance in order to relieve withdrawal symptoms.

2. At least some of the symptoms associated with the problems have lasted a minimum of one month or problems have recurred over longer periods of time.

Psychoactive substance dependence is classified according to its severity (i.e., mild, moderate, or severe) and whether it has been in partial remission (the condition is somewhat better) or full remission (the condition is much better). The type of substance that is the focus of the problem is indicated. There are ten general classes of substances. It is not uncommon, however, that an individual may use multiple substances. As noted earlier, we will primarily focus on (1) alcohol and (2) sedative, hypnotic, and anxiolytic drugs. Sedatives are drugs used to calm or quiet the individual, hypnotics are primarily used to induce sleep, and anxiolytics (also called anti-anxiety drugs) help to reduce anxiety.

Another classification of substance use problems is made by *DSM-III-R:* psychoactive substance *abuse.* This disorder refers to use of a substance (or substances) that causes any of a variety of social, psychological, occupational, or health problems but for which difficulties are not as severe or pervasive as those outlined in psychoactive substance dependence.

Frequency

It appears that about 6 percent of older people living in the community (that is, living outside of institutions) engage in "heavy drinking." Probably only 1–2 percent, however, meet criteria for substance abuse or dependence—rates much lower than those found among younger individuals. Men are at greater risk for alcohol problems than are women. Older adults with alcohol problems have sometimes been divided into early- versus late-onset alcoholics. About two-thirds of older adults with alcohol problems developed those problems earlier in life. For a minority, however, alcohol-related difficulties had their onset in the later years.

Most studies have found that drug abuse (that is, nonalcohol substance abuse) and dependence, as defined by standardized psychiatric criteria, are almost nonexistent in older adults. This stands in stark contrast to research that indicates that older adults are heavy users of sedatives, hypnotics, or anxiolytics. One study, for example, found that almost one-quarter of older adults reported using psychoactive drugs prescribed by their physician in the previous year. The apparent low prevalence of drug abuse and dependence among older adults also stands in contrast to research that has found that older people often do not take medications in the manner in which they are prescribed. Some mental health professionals have suggested that there is widespread "misuse" of prescribed and over-the-counter medications by older persons, and, as noted earlier, some believe that there is widespread overprescribing of psychoactive medications to the elderly by physicians. Misuse of drugs by the elderly is the focus of some current research and, in the coming years, a better understanding of this apparent problem will be available.

Possible Causes

There are a variety of social, psychological, and biological theories about why individuals develop alcohol-related problems. Although the theories about why significant problems develop in late life are less well developed, late-life stressors may play an important role. For example, retirement, loss of friends or spouse, or physical illness may lead to increased alcohol consumption and risk for alcohol dependency. Widespread availability of alcohol and its frequent use in reducing stress contributes to the risk for alcoholism.

Frances Carlson's neighbor alerted the social service outreach worker to the fact that Mrs. Carlson had had a series of "accidents" in recent months, as a result of which she might need help. She also confided that she had seen Mrs. Carlson "staggering" down the hallway one night and suspected that Mrs. Carlson had been drinking too much lately.

Mrs. Carlson was receptive to a visit by the outreach worker. During the course of the visit, she pointed out a large bruise on her right arm that she said was caused by a fan that "fell" on her. She mentioned several other "accidents" but dismissed them, saying she was "accident prone." Mrs. Carlson did admit, however, that she had had problems adjusting since she retired the previous year. "My work was my life. What is my life now?" she remarked. She lamented the fact that she did not have grandchildren and said that her daughter had died in adolescence and her husband had died when she was in her fifties. She noted that most of her friends from work had moved away from the area. Asked if she was a drinker, Mrs. Carlson laughed and said, "All my life." Later on, she confessed that perhaps she had been drinking more than usual and that this might not be the best thing.

Mrs. Carlson was referred to a social worker who engaged her in brief psychotherapy. The social worker also helped Mrs. Carlson to move to subsidized senior citizen housing and to take part in a community group for older people. The social worker later told the outreach worker that Mrs. Carlson indeed had had a serious drinking problem since retirement, but that she was responsive to opportunities that had been offered to her for social contact with peers. In recent months she appeared much happier and apparently had stopped drinking.

Some specific risk factors for alcoholism in late life include a life history of regular drinking, certain personality styles (mainly the tendency to be anxious and worrisome), and interpersonal losses. Alcoholism may also be a response to psychiatric difficulties. Some individuals, for example, consume alcohol to relieve feelings of depression—although in the long run alcohol will make the depression worse. In addition, some individuals seem to have a genetic vulnerability to alcoholism, although this does not appear to be a factor among those for whom alcohol-related problems begin in late life.

Drug dependence, abuse, and misuse probably have multiple origins. Several possibilities have been suggested by geriatric psychiatrist Dan Blazer: poor communication between patient and doctor, the patient's failure to comply with instructions for taking medications, the sharing and swapping of medications among the elderly, abuse of over-the-counter drugs, and the "do something" tendency of doctors to prescribe unnecessary medication. The last refers to prescribing medications, particularly sedative, hypnotic, and anxiolytic drugs, to meet the patient's or the doctor's expectation that "something should be done" even though the patient's condition does not meet conventionally accepted standards for prescribing the particular medication.

Evaluation

Drug and alcohol problems may go undetected for many years. Shame and embarrassment often surround their use and both the older person with a substance use problem and family members may try to minimize its significance. Health care providers may also feel reluctant to confront an older patient with the possibility that he or she is substance abusing or substance dependent. Also, some of the reasons that younger alcoholics come to the attention of mental health professionals are less common among older individuals. For example, alcoholism may interfere with a younger individual's capacity to engage in competitive employment, thereby creating serious financial problems that may motivate the individual to seek help. Many older people are retired, however, and the socially damaging effects of alcoholism may be easier to disguise. A careful diagnostic evaluation of substance abuse and dependence is important, however, since prolonged use has been associated with an array of medical, psychological, and social problems.

Most older people metabolize alcohol differently from younger persons. Most notably, older persons need less alcohol to achieve the same blood alcohol level as younger individuals. Given the less efficient functioning of various organ systems in older people, consumption of large amounts of alcohol can tax the body by, for example, irritating the intestinal system (with subsequent constipation or diarrhea), accumulating fatty substances in the liver, and increasing urine flow (which may aggravate prostate problems in men).

A good diagnostic work-up for alcohol problems requires an accurate assessment of the amount of alcohol that the individual actually uses. This information may not be easy to obtain since, like younger persons with alcohol problems, the older individual may minimize his or her alcohol intake. Information from sources other than the older alcoholic may be critical to gain a more complete picture of the problem. Since chronic alcohol use is associated with physical health problems, a medical work-up is most important. The longer-term consequences of alcoholism may include impairment of the heart, liver, intestinal system, and pancreas and may also result in nutritional deficiencies and sleep disturbances. The older individual's cognitive abilities should also be evaluated. Chronic alcoholism may cause neurological impairment, most notably Wernicke-Korsakoff's syndrome. Wernicke-Korsakoff's syndrome is a type of dementia that develops in alcoholics because of nutritional deficiency (the lack of vitamin B-12) and direct damage to the brain caused by the alcohol. Problematic personal and interpersonal relationships are frequently seen among alcoholics, and an assessment of the social resources that may or may not be available to the older individual should be done. Psychiatric symptoms, including depression, anxiety, psychosis, and delirium, must be evaluated since they may accompany alcoholism.

Although nonalcohol substance dependence appears to be rare in the older population, drug misuse is probably more common. Dependence on sedatives, hypnotics, and anxiolytics is probably the most common type of drug problem in older adults. Given the frequency with which these drugs are prescribed to older individuals, dependency on one or several of them (obtained through legitimate prescriptions from their physicians) may develop over time. Development of toxicity from these medications may alert the mental health professional that the older person has a drug problem. As has been discussed previously, drug toxicity may cause symptoms of delirium or reversible dementia. Dependence on these medications may come to the attention of the health professional only when the individual is hospitalized for an unrelated condition. Deprived of usual access to these medications, the individual may begin to evidence symptoms of withdrawal. Withdrawal from sedatives, hypnotics, or anxiolytics (as well as from alcohol) must be managed carefully since withdrawal symptoms are sometimes life threatening. As with other conditions, a good history of past and current mental health difficulties must be taken and medical, psychiatric, and psychosocial evaluations are also needed.

Treatment

The older alcoholic may initially need to be detoxified. This may require hospitalization, although sometimes it can be done on an outpatient basis. The goal of treatment is to help the individual, once detoxified, to abstain from alcohol and to develop better personal and social resources to cope with daily life. Some physicians prescribe the drug disulfiram (trade name Antabuse) to assist the individual in abstaining from alcohol. If the person consumes alcohol while taking disulfiram, a variety of unpleasant symptoms will ensue (e.g., headaches, nausea, and vomiting). Although some have argued that disulfiram is safe for the elderly, others have advised that this medication should be prescribed with caution, especially for elderly with physical health problems. The family of the older alcoholic must be enlisted in treatment and alerted to the potentially serious consequences of continued alcohol use. Some mental health professionals have found that older individuals are more comfortable in alcohol rehabilitation programs that are specifically designed for older people than in mixed-age programs. Alcoholics Anonymous (AA)–sponsored groups may be useful for older adults, especially those with tenuous social ties. AA groups may form the nucleus around which a system of supportive relationships is developed with others who share the same problem.

Older adults with nonalcohol drug dependence problems may need to be hospitalized if they are showing signs of toxicity from sedatives, hypnotics, or anxiolytics. Hospitalization is also sometimes useful to assist the individual in withdrawing from these drugs. Subsequent education about the dangers of drug misuse and abuse may be most helpful since many individuals may not have fully understood the potential danger of these drugs. Family monitoring of the older person's medication may be important, particularly if the older individual continues to try to obtain drugs. If life stresses have precipitated misuse, abuse, or dependence on psychiatric medications, the individual may profit by a problem-oriented psychotherapy to help him or her to better cope with later life stresses.

Outcome of Substance Use Disorders in Late Life

In view of the fact that alcoholics have higher rates of mortality than nonalcoholics, the consequences of failing to receive treatment may be dire. Different therapeutic approaches appear to hold promise for successful treatment of both alcohol and drug problems. In general, older alcoholics appear to do as well in alcohol rehabilitation programs as younger persons do, although some have found that those with later-onset alcoholism have a better prognosis for successful treatment than individuals with lifelong alcohol problems. Despite current belief, there is no available research that indicates that age-segregated alcohol rehabilitation programs are more effective than age-integrated programs. There are no studies that have carefully evaluated the usefulness of treatments for sedative, hypnotic, or anxiolytic misuse, abuse, or dependence in later life. Based on their own professional experience, however, some well-established geriatric mental health professionals report that older people improve in response to efforts to treat these drug problems.

Chapter 4

The Mental Health System and the Older Adult

BASIC FACTS

- Historically the mentally ill have not been treated well by their societies. Older adults with mental health problems appear to have fared particularly badly.

- Until the 1960s large numbers of people with serious mental disorders were resident in state psychiatric institutions. As many as one-third of these residents were people age 65 or older.

- In part because of concerns about the negative effects of institutional environments on the mentally ill, many patients were discharged in the 1960s and 1970s. Adequate community care was not subsequently provided for many of these individuals.

- Many elderly patients discharged from state institutions became residents of nursing homes—places that did not have the resources to adequately address the mental health needs of their older residents.

- The current system of outpatient mental health care for older adults includes private practitioners, community mental health centers and mental health clinics, health maintenance organizations, the Department of Veterans Affairs (VA) clinics, and social service organizations.

145

- The current system of inpatient care includes short-term ("acute") hospitals and long-term care facilities.

- Funding for mental health services for older adults primarily comes from state monies and federal support in the form of Medicare and Medicaid.

- Identified problems in providing care to older people in the current system of mental health care include: (1) inadequate financing, (2) lack of training and manpower, (3) poor coordination among service systems, and (4) reluctance of some older adults to use mental health services.

Introduction

Despite its limitations, the existing knowledge base on the prevalence, nature, and treatment of mental disorders in the older adult is a valuable resource on which both professionals and the general public may draw. It is the accumulated knowledge of years of research and clinical work that provides guidance for current practice and points the way for further advances. This may be little comfort, however, for individuals unable to locate or afford competently delivered mental health services.

It is important to communicate at the outset that there is general dissatisfaction with the existing system of mental health care for older adults. The system is generally characterized as underfunded, "fragmented," and underutilized by the older adults who need care most. Most mental health problems actually come to the attention of general practitioners (that is, family medical doctors), who are often unfamiliar with mental health issues and too often misdiagnose and inadequately treat mental disorders in the elderly. Even many mental health professionals are unfamiliar with the unique problems of older adults and are unaware of current developments in the field of mental health and aging. There is a shortage of well-trained geriatric mental health specialists—a shortage that will become more acute as the number of elderly within the U.S. population grows.

This chapter will address several questions about the existing mental health system for older adults:

What is the history of mental health care for the aged?

What constitutes the current system of mental health care for older adults?

How do financial and reimbursement issues affect the availability and quality of mental health care for older adults?

What are the major problems that currently exist within the mental health care system for older adults?

How can mental health services for older adults be found?

How can older persons and their families be knowledgeable consumers of mental health services?

Historical Perspectives on Care of Older Adults with Mental Disorders

Historically, people with mental disorders have not been treated well by their societies. In part, societies' responses to the mentally ill have reflected the way they view mental illness. In Europe of the Middle Ages, mental disorders were seen as evidence of witchcraft or "the devil's work," for which the individual bore responsibility. Society's response was to punish the mentally ill; punishment included death by execution. In the seventeenth and eighteenth centuries, the mentally ill within Europe were regarded as unfortunates who were reluctantly provided with the most rudimentary of material support.

In the early history of the United States, financially destitute mentally ill persons were "auctioned off" by some communities to the lowest bidders, who promised to provide for their physical care. As cities grew, institutions developed (actually poorhouses) for the "care" of the mentally ill and other social undesirables. The nineteenth century witnessed the development of "moral treatment," a relatively enlightened approach to mental illness. Moral treatment was a sort of occupational therapy that redirected the individual from so-called self-absorption to active involvement with the larger community. These efforts were thought to have the potential for curing mental illness. During this era, however, most mentally ill people continued to be confined to poorhouses, and eventually even institutions founded on the principles of moral treatment became simply custodial. The particular fate of the elderly with mental disorders in distant history is not generally known. Some research has suggested that even when some attempt was made to actually help the mentally ill, the elderly were unlikely to be the recipients of these efforts because they were seen as less likely to benefit from them than younger persons.

By the first half of the twentieth century, the number and size of psychiatric institutions had grown significantly. In the mid-1950s there were more than half a million individuals residing in state, county, city, private, and veterans mental institutions. From one-quarter to one-third of the residents were people 65 years or older. The large percentage of elderly residents was, in part, a function of low rates of discharge from the institutions (i.e., people came, stayed, and "aged in place") and of the fact that there were large numbers of people with dementia in the institutions. Since the mid-1950s, however, the population of mental institutions has declined dramatically. This change reflected several factors. The introduction of anti-psychotic medications significantly controlled psychotic symptoms and increased the likelihood that many individuals could reside outside of institutions. Many leading mental health care professionals argued that large-scale institutionalization was harmful since it eventually eroded existing self-care skills of residents. Most states found the cost of running mental institutions burdensome and welcomed the opportunity to discharge patients, thereby saving money and also appearing socially progressive.

In 1963, President John F. Kennedy proposed the development of a nationwide, comprehensive system of care for the mentally ill. He urged the development of 1,500 community mental health centers (CMHCs). Five types of "essential" services would be the foundation of CMHCs: (1) inpatient care, (2) outpatient care, (3) emergency care, (4) partial hospitalization, and (5) mental health consultation and education. In addition, five other types of services would be offered as resources: (1) diagnostic services, (2) rehabilitation services, (3) pre-care and aftercare, (4) training, and (5) research and evaluation. Each

CMHC would serve a geographically defined region called a catchment area, which would be small enough so that all citizens would receive competent care within no more than 45 minutes' driving time. CMHCs were seen as serving all residents regardless of age, income, or race. The federal government would provide "seed" money to CMHCs to begin operation, and then those federal monies would be phased out as CMHCs became self-supporting by collecting a variety of public mental health and private insurance monies from the patients they served. A bold vision for humane treatment of people with mental disorders, CMHCs began to be developed in the mid-1960s. Unfortunately, the vision was never realized and unanticipated problems followed early efforts to change the mental health care system.

Only one-third of the originally proposed CMHCs were actually developed. Existing CMHCs found it difficult to become financially self-sustaining after federal monies were withdrawn. Many CMHCs began to increasingly serve less advantaged individuals, many of whom had multiple needs. Those with financial resources that included private insurance reimbursement (originally foreseen as an important source of revenue for CMHCs) turned to other sectors for mental health care. Although it was thought that deinstitutionalization of patients would free monies that could then be used for community mental health care, this did not happen.

The problems surrounding deinstitutionalization of psychiatric hospitals in the 1960s and 1970s and attempts to develop community services were complex. In essence, however, people were deinstitutionalized but CMHCs and other community services were never able to meet many of the deinstitutionalized patients' needs. This was in part because: (1) some deinstitutionalized individuals actually needed custodial care; (2) as noted, CMHCs were not adequately funded and only a fraction of the projected number were actually developed; (3) there was an enormous demand for low-cost housing by discharged patients that was not readily met; and (4) despite the philosophy that individuals would be happier living and receiving services within their own communities, some patients did not feel that they had communities to which they could return. As well, some of their communities did not welcome mental patients.

What happened to elderly residents of psychiatric institutions? Many of them were discharged to nursing homes or board and care facilities (also called residential care facilities—residences that provide food, housing, and minimal support), which were generally unprepared to deal with mental health problems. There were, however, clear financial incentives to many states to move older individuals from state institutions into nursing homes. The federal program of health insurance for the poor, Medicaid, paid for residence in nursing homes but not for care in state institutions. Even though states share in the cost of Medicaid, many anticipated considerable savings by moving older people into nursing homes.

What about the role of CMHCs in providing mental health care services to older adults? It is generally acknowledged that most CMHCs have not adequately addressed the needs of the older individuals in their catchment area. The evidence for this, in part, comes from the failure of many older adults to utilize services from CMHCs. At present, older adults only utilize 5–6 percent of CMHC services (some estimates are as low as 1–2 percent) although they make up approximately 11 percent of the population. Most feel that the underutilization of the CMHC system is not the fault of individual CMHCs, but rather lies in governmental mental health policies that offer few incentives for the delivery of mental health care to older adults. There have been repeated calls in the last ten years for policy changes to make CMHCs more responsive to the needs of older adults, but these calls have generally gone unheeded. CMHCs are not alone, however, in their inability to provide comprehensive care to older adults. Problems exist throughout the system (or what one author refers to as the nonsystem) of mental health care for the aged.

The Present System of Mental Health Care for Older Adults

As discussed in previous chapters, mental health care is generally obtained either on an outpatient or inpatient basis. The latter is usually differentiated on the basis of whether the treatment is acute (that is, short-term) or custodial (long-term).

Outpatient Mental Health Care

Interestingly, about half of older adults do not receive outpatient mental health care from mental health professionals. They receive such services from community physicians, to whom older adults frequently bring their emotional as well as their medical problems. As noted earlier, there is concern about the quality of diagnosis and treatment provided by community physicians to older adults with mental disorders.

The formal system of mental health care includes (1) private practitioners of mental health services; (2) publicly funded services, primarily CMHCs and hospital-based clinics; (3) health maintenance organizations (HMOs); (4) hospitals and clinics operated by the Department of Veterans Affairs; and (5) other community agencies that, among a variety of services, offer mental health care.

PRIVATE MENTAL HEALTH CARE

Some mental health professionals provide services on a private, fee-for-service basis to older adults. The fees of mental health professionals vary according to the type of professional (psychiatrists typically charge more than others), the experience and reputation of the service provider (more experienced professionals usually charge more than the less experienced), and the geographical area (services provided in more urbanized areas are usually more costly than those in rural areas). Utilization of private mental health services by the elderly is rare—estimates range from 0 percent to 3.3 percent. Although there is a paucity of research on the use of private mental health services by the aged, it is likely that many professionals who deliver such services have had little training in the treatment of late-life mental health problems. An important contributing factor to low rates of use of private care is likely Medicare's historically limited reimbursement for private outpatient mental health services.

PUBLIC MENTAL HEALTH CARE

As discussed earlier, individual CMHCs offer services to individuals residing in their catchment areas. Problems in utilization of these services by older adults were addressed earlier. Many

CMHCs offer a range of mental health services that are usually provided on an ability-to-pay basis. A few CMHCs offer specialized services for older adults. Another source of mental health care is outpatient clinics housed in public and private hospitals. Most of these mental health clinics offer services to people of all ages, although the number of specialized geriatric mental health clinics is slowly increasing. One advantage of hospital-based mental health clinics is that Medicare has historically reimbursed such services more generously than outpatient services obtained in other sectors.

HEALTH MAINTENANCE ORGANIZATIONS (HMOs)

HMOs are organizations that usually provide a package of outpatient and inpatient medical services. They are often comprehensive health plans that require only small out-of-pocket fees for services that are used. To contain costs, HMOs try to carefully monitor use of services. Most HMOs provide some mental health care but usually do so only because these services are mandated by state or federal laws. HMOs typically limit the number of outpatient mental health visits or inpatient days that will be provided as part of the plan. HMOs therefore are generally seen as offering limited options for people with mental disorders.

DEPARTMENT OF VETERANS AFFAIRS SERVICES

The Department of Veterans Affairs (VA) operates outpatient clinics and many other health services throughout the country. Many clinics offer mental health care and some of them offer specialized mental health services for the older veteran. With the large number of World War II veterans who are now older adults, the VA has been faced with providing health and mental health care to an increasingly large geriatric population. Eligibility for VA health services has generally been restricted to certain subgroups of veterans; those with other health care options are encouraged to use them and not the VA system.

OTHER SOURCES OF MENTAL HEALTH CARE

Some community agencies provide a range of services that include mental health care and, occasionally, services for older adults. For example, affiliates of Family Service America all provide counseling services and sometimes offer specialized services for older adults. In addition, the philanthropic arms of the major religious organizations in this country support a variety of community services, some of which include services for older people with mental health difficulties.

It is important to mention that the above discussion uses a fairly strict definition of mental health services. Some older individuals with mental disorders may require, in addition to diagnosis and treatment, supportive services (for example, transportation, delivered meals, home-care services, or recreational services), the availability of which varies locally and regionally. Area Agencies on Aging—organizations that are federally mandated to oversee services outlined in the Older Americans Act—often coordinate such services. People with dementia, in particular, may be in need of home support services, adult day programs, respite care, and related kinds of help. The need of people with mental disorders for multiple services, in fact, is not always well addressed by mental and nonmental health care systems.

Inpatient Mental Health Services

ACUTE (SHORT-TERM) HOSPITALIZATION

Most inpatient hospitalization for mental health difficulties actually takes place within general hospitals (not psychiatric hospitals), with most services provided by nonpsychiatrist physicians. Some general hospitals, however, have specialized psychiatric units that are more likely to provide core mental health services such as psychotherapy, psychopharmacology, and recreational rehabilitation. In contrast, psychiatric hospitals are exclusively devoted to the care of mental disorders. They may be part of medical centers or may operate independently (these are referred to as free-standing hospitals), sometimes as for-profit businesses. Psychiatric hospitals usually provide the most comprehensive inpatient mental health care. As noted earlier, CMHCs offer inpatient services for those in need of short-term, or acute, hospitalization. State psychiatric institutions and VA facilities often offer acute hospitalization in addition to longer-term inpatient care. Few institutions have specialized geriatric inpatient mental health services.

LONG-TERM CARE

Although older adults once constituted more than one-quarter of
the population of state psychiatric hospitals, they now compose
only a small percentage. Occasionally some long-term (custodial) care is provided to older adults in the state hospital system,
but for the most part, such care is now provided in nursing
homes and board and care facilities. In essence, the nursing home
has taken the place of the state hospital in caring for older people
with chronic mental disorders. In fact, mental illness is common
among elderly residents of nursing homes. Older people with
mental disorders residing in nursing homes include not only
those who were previously residents of state psychiatric hospitals, but also those who directly entered the nursing home system
from the community because of mental disorders and those who
developed mental health problems after nursing home admis-
sion. It is generally agreed that the quality of mental health care
in nursing homes and similar facilities is poor. Such facilities
usually do not have onsite personnel or programs to adequately
deal with the mental health needs of their residents.

The Funding of Mental Health
Care for Older Adults

Individual states provide the bulk of funding for mental health
care by supporting a network of inpatient and outpatient facilities. The federal government pays for most of the remaining costs
of mental health care, with a small percentage paid by private
insurance. The federal government channels most of its support
for mental health care through Medicaid, the medical insurance
program for the indigent that is funded by both the federal
government and states. Medicare only pays a negligible amount
of mental health care costs.

Medicare

Since its creation, Medicare has maintained clear restrictions on
its reimbursement of mental health services. These restrictions
include payment limits for most outpatient and inpatient services

and a lack of freedom to choose the kind of mental health professional one desires (i.e., Medicare primarily reimburses services provided by M.D.s). At the time of this writing, a number of issues related to Medicare reimbursement for health and mental health services are being debated within the Congress, and the likely outcome of this debate remains unclear. We will therefore only offer an overview of Medicare's support of mental health services for older adults. The reader is urged to contact a local Social Security office for the most up-to-date information on reimbursement of mental health services.

Historically, Medicare has severely restricted the amount that it would pay for outpatient mental health services delivered by private (mental health) practitioners (which basically meant M.D.s). It did this by requiring a 50 percent co-payment of "reasonable charges" for mental health services (in contrast to 20 percent co-payment for medical expenses) and by limiting the total amount that would be paid for mental health services each year. For 20 years, the amount that would be reimbursed was $250, but this was raised to $1,100 for 1989. Starting in July 1990 there will be no limit on reimbursement, although a 50 percent co-payment will continue to be required. Another important change that will be effective July 1990 is that most services provided by psychologists and some services provided by social workers will also be covered.

Outpatient mental health services offered in hospital settings, however, have been reimbursed more liberally by Medicare. In hospital settings there have not been restrictions on the amount that would be paid for outpatient coverage each year and such services only required a 20 percent co-payment. In contrast, there have been restrictions on payments for services provided in CMHCs. In recent years, more generous reimbursement has been provided for the payment of some expenses associated with the diagnosis and treatment of dementia.

Medicare has a total cap of 190 days of inpatient care that will be paid for in a psychiatric hospital. Somewhat more liberal rules have applied, however, for some types of psychiatric care delivered in a general hospital. It is not surprising, therefore, that Medicare payments for mental health services only account for 2–3 percent of all Medicare expenses.

In an attempt to control health care costs, in 1983 Medicare instituted a "prospective payment system" whereby hospitals were paid based on the average number of days of hospitalization deemed necessary for a particular diagnosis (these determinations are known as diagnosis-related groups or DRGs). This was in contrast to the previous payment system, in which hospitals were reimbursed for all costs incurred in patient care. A temporary exemption to these rules was made for psychiatric hospitals and psychiatric units of general hospitals because of problems in the development of DRGs for psychiatric diagnoses. The psychiatric profession has generally resisted efforts to apply DRGs to psychiatric problems, arguing that it is extremely difficult to calculate an average number of days of hospitalization for psychiatric diagnoses since patient needs vary considerably within each diagnostic classification. The future of psychiatric DRGs is still being debated.

Medicaid

Medicaid is the federal program that provides matching funds to states to cover medical care for the indigent. Some estimates are that Medicaid covers almost one-quarter of all health care costs in this country and comprises two-thirds of federal funding of mental health. Since states share in the cost of Medicaid, rules governing coverage of health services vary from state to state. Coverage of mental health care by Medicaid has usually been more comprehensive than that offered by Medicare. Medicare is often used in conjunction with Medicaid when an older person, by virtue of low income, qualifies for Medicaid. In many states Medicaid covers the cost of outpatient and inpatient mental health services without the kinds of restrictions imposed by Medicare. What Medicaid is willing to pay for these services, however, is often less than that paid by other health insurers. As a result, there is a disincentive for some individuals or organizations to provide services to Medicaid recipients.

Medicaid pays for almost half of all nursing home costs in this country. It is worth noting that although the de facto mental health policy has been to place older people with mental disorders in nursing homes, in many states Medicaid will not fund nursing homes that are predominantly populated by persons with mental disorders. The rationale for this is that provision of mental health services is primarily the responsibility of individual states and not of the federal government. As a consequence, there is an incentive for nursing homes to minimize the reported prevalence of mental disorders among their residents. This practice has, in part, contributed to a widespread failure to diagnose and treat mental health problems in nursing homes since some nursing homes would lose Medicaid funding if the true prevalence of mental health problems among their residents were known.

Private Insurance

For people of all age groups, private insurance coverage of mental health services is more limited than for physical health services. For older adults, private health insurance coverage of mental health services is extremely limited. Although there are plans offered by insurance companies to supplement Medicare coverage (so-called Medi-gap plans), they rarely cover mental health services.

Problems in the Mental Health Care System for Older Adults

As implied by the foregoing discussion, there are many problems in the delivery of mental health services to older adults. These include problems with (1) financing, (2) training and manpower, (3) coordinating among service systems, and (4) reaching older persons who have mental health problems. The unmet needs of nursing home residents well illustrate the many problems of providing mental health care to older people.

Financial Problems

Medicare was designed with clear disincentives for older people's use of outpatient mental health services. Although most individuals with mental health problems would not exhaust Medicare's limited number of days of inpatient services provided in a psychiatric hospital, this restriction could be extremely burdensome for those with severe difficulties that require frequent hospitalizations. It is of interest that the catastrophic health care bill passed in 1988 and then rescinded in 1989 retained the limit on inpatient care in a psychiatric hospital that would be paid for by Medicare.

While Medicaid has usually been more generous than Medicare in funding mental health services for older people, only the financially destitute are eligible for Medicaid. Ironically, while many Medicaid recipients in nursing homes are most in need of mental health services, they are unlikely to receive them. As noted before, Medicare has generally maintained a policy against funding settings that are predominately populated by persons with mental health problems.

Training and Manpower Problems

There is a lack of mental health professionals (including psychiatrists, psychologists, nurses, and social workers) with training in mental health and aging. Since the mental health needs of older adults have historically been ignored it comes as little surprise that few professionals are trained to address those needs. There have also been few professional incentives to specialize in the delivery of mental health services to the aged since working with the aged has carried little prestige.

As health policy planners and policymakers began to reckon with the expanding population of older adults in the United States, it became apparent that the physical and mental health needs of older people would eventually outstrip available manpower. In the last ten years important strides have been made to promote the development of specialized geriatric training programs for health and mental health professionals and retraining programs for those wishing to respecialize in geriatrics. The fact remains, however, that it will take many years to recruit and train the number of professionals required to service the growing need for specialized physical and mental health services for the aged. Some have suggested that, because community physicians provide the bulk of mental health care for older adults, efforts should be made to better educate them about issues in mental health and aging.

Coordination Problems among Service Systems

The various components of the health and mental health care system are not usually well coordinated. Multiple service systems, often funded by different sources and varying in their knowledge of and interest in coordinating with other systems, create what is sometimes referred to as service fragmentation. To add to the problem, within each system there may be several subsystems. As noted, in the mental health field there are public, private, outpatient, acute inpatient, and long-term care services. Coordination of services within such a mental health system may be difficult. Coordinating among several systems (or among several subsystems within systems) is a formidable task. The result is that sometimes people in need of specific services, in common parlance, fall between the cracks.

Older adults are particularly vulnerable to service fragmentation since they often have multiple needs. For example, consider an older individual with serious cardiac problems who has a major depression. As a consequence of these conditions, the individual cannot adequately care for him- or herself. The individual may need inpatient and outpatient medical care (involving several medical doctors), mental health care, home-care services (perhaps delivered meals or a home health aide), and possibly transportation to medical and mental health outpatient appointments. Who coordinates these activities? Family members often take active roles. But family members are sometimes unfamiliar with the complexities of the service system and must learn "on the job." If the older individual is fortunate, a professional, typically a social worker, will coordinate the delivery of services (an activity called case management). In large urban areas, where service systems may constitute large bureaucracies, service coordination is particularly problematic. People with mental disorders may face additional difficulties as well. Some organizations may be reluctant to provide nonmental health services to older people with mental disorders for fear that they may be "difficult" clients. Also, nonmental health providers may not appropriately refer their clients with mental disorders for mental health care.

Some states have made serious efforts to improve service coordination by establishing agency linkages, by working more closely with Area Agencies on Aging, by offering special reimbursement rates that reward interagency cooperation, and by developing intra- and interagency education programs on the mental health needs of older adults.

Older People's Reluctance To Use Services

Some older people may resist using mental health services even when those service are made readily available. As noted in earlier chapters, some older people view use of mental health services as a stigma because they lived their younger years when considerable shame was attached to having mental health problems. Some older people are also aware that the preferred mode of treatment for serious mental disorders in the past was incarceration in large state psychiatric hospitals. Some mental health providers have, in fact, noted that the reluctance of some older persons to go for evaluation and treatment of mental health problems is a result of their fear that receiving mental health services is the first step toward institutionalization.

Most older people tend to be fairly independent. They have lived their lives with some measure of success, coped with the wide variety of difficulties that life usually presents, and feel that they can contend with the problems of late life. Even if an individual acknowledges that he or she is having problems, the suggestion that mental health services are needed may be viewed as offensive. Consequently, it is small wonder that, if given a choice, many older individuals would bring their mental health problems to their physicians instead of to a mental health professional. Some mental health professionals have suggested that, if properly educated, many community physicians might be able to provide reasonably good basic mental health services for older adults. In view of the trust that many older persons place in their doctors, community physicians are at the very least in a good position to make referrals to mental health professionals.

Although many family members of older people with mental disorders, especially adult children, do not hold significant negative conceptions about mental health care, they may not be aware that effective treatments exist for many mental disorders. In the case of dementia, family members may attribute cognitive changes to old age and feel that nothing can be done. Or, while aware that the older person has a dementia, they may fail to realize that services sometimes exist to help the family manage the dementia patient.

Ultimately, it is the responsibility of the mental health care system to design services that take into account the concerns of older people and their families. In an ideal system, mental health services would be provided in a variety of settings that are easily accessible and nonstigmatizing.

Problems in Nursing Homes

The majority of persons residing in nursing homes appear to have mental health problems. Estimates range from 35–85 percent. More than half of nursing home residents have dementia. Most older nursing home residents with mental health problems do not, however, receive mental health services. One study of the mental health needs of nursing home residents, for example, found that only 15 percent of those who needed such services actually received them. As discussed earlier, an important reason for this unmet need is a reimbursement system that discourages diagnosis and treatment of mental disorders in nursing home residents.

There are other problems. In many cases nursing home staff are poorly trained to deal with the myriad and complex emotional and behavioral problems of nursing home residents. Dementia patients may present particularly formidable behavioral problems including screaming, crying, spitting, wandering off, and assaulting staff or other residents. A frequent response to such behaviors is prescribing neuroleptic (anti-psychotic) medications. Unfortunately, these medications are frequently misprescribed or are not carefully monitored and can, in some cases, actually exacerbate the problems they are supposed to improve. Access of nursing home residents to psychological treatment, such as psychotherapy, is extremely limited. Psychotherapy could potentially be very beneficial in helping some residents with mental disorders, with problems in adaptation to the nursing home environment, death and dying issues, and other concerns. Psychologists would be particularly well suited to do this kind of work. Only a few nursing homes in the country, however, employ psychologists.

Nursing homes face problems in the recruitment and retention of competent staff. Some nursing home personnel, from administrators to orderlies, experience considerable frustration in doing their work given the limited resources that are usually available. Anger, hostility, disappointment, disillusionment, and other symptoms characteristic of what has been called burnout make the provision of humane care a formidable challenge.

Practical Suggestions for Finding and Using Mental Health Services

The foregoing discussion may leave the reader wondering if it is possible to find mental health services for older people. The answer is a qualified yes. The problems in the mental health system are detailed not to dissuade people from pursuing such services but partly as a caveat that the existing system does not easily accommodate the needs of older people. Many people reasonably expect that a well-integrated system of mental health care exists for older adults; they may feel considerable frustration and even anger upon discovering that it does not. It is more likely that needed services will be found if an individual is armed with the facts and a reasonably well thought out plan for obtaining care.

It is important to emphasize that there are a growing number of well-qualified, dedicated, concerned geriatric mental health professionals. Fairly well integrated and coordinated systems of mental health care exist in some areas. Many persons are working at all levels of government to improve the funding and delivery of mental health services for older adults. Persons directing mental health care systems are often painfully aware of inadequacies. Similarly, many people providing direct mental health and related services to older adults are distressed when options are limited for providing help. Increasing numbers of persons with mental disorders and their families are lobbying for better research and services. Things are slowly improving.

How To Find Services

The resource section of this book lists a variety of organizations that may be of help in locating mental health services for older adults. This information will provide a number of clues in the detective work of finding mental health services. If an older person appears to need mental health assistance, however, several questions need to be answered at the outset. Have problems reached crisis proportions so that help is needed immediately? For example, is the older adult in danger of harming him- or herself or others? Some persons are in real danger of trying to commit suicide or are so seriously confused or disoriented that they could unintentionally harm themselves if left alone. Other individuals may become so aggressive that they may be in danger of assaulting those around them. In circumstances like these, immediate attention is required. It may be necessary to take the individual to a hospital emergency room, arrange for an immediate evaluation by the family physician, or, in dire circumstances, call the police. Although these are rare circumstances, they must be dealt with immediately.

More typically, problems develop more slowly and there is time to check out the availability of local mental health services. Where to start depends on where one resides. Some areas have a variety of agencies and individuals, both public and private, that offer mental health services. Service options are more likely to exist in urban areas. In rural areas services are usually more limited.

The family physician may be the first person you should check with for a referral to public or private mental health services.

The local general hospital or medical center may have mental health services or know where such services might be found.

Ministers, priests, or rabbis may know of mental health resources. Some religious organizations raise funds for support of community services that sometimes include mental health care for the aged.

Community mental health centers may sometimes be located by looking in the telephone book under this name, or it may be helpful to look under "mental health clinics" or "hospitals" in the Yellow Pages.

State departments of mental health or mental hygiene may offer assistance in locating local mental health resources.

Area Agencies on Aging, the government-funded local organizations that help coordinate services for older persons, often have information and referral services.

Some community organizations have personnel with mental health training or even specialized training in mental health and aging.

For persons with dementia, a slowly increasing number of day programs, respite care programs, and, for the caregiver, support programs are being offered through a variety of organizations.

University-affiliated hospitals and medical centers may be particularly good places to find geriatric mental health specialty clinics. Some universities and medical centers sponsor geriatric psychiatry fellowship programs that offer advanced training for psychiatrists interested in specializing in mental health and aging. Many of these programs offer excellent psychiatric care for older people with mental disorders.

The VA operates a large network of inpatient and outpatient health and mental health care facilities that are available to some veterans. Of note are the Department of Veterans Affairs' Geriatric Research, Education, and Clinical Centers (GRECCs). Some of these offer specialized mental health services for older veterans.

The resource section of this book lists some governmental, professional, and self-help/advocacy organizations that may be able to provide information about mental health problems as well as assistance in locating local mental health resources. For people with dementia and their families, the Alzheimer's Association sponsors local chapters and support groups throughout the country that can provide up-to-date information about dementia and local resources. Self-help/advocacy groups for people with mental illness and their families exist throughout the country. They may offer leads in locating mental health resources.

Although in the past these self-help groups have not focused on the problems of older adults, some of them evidence interest in doing so in the future.

How To Use Mental Health Services

Many people view health care as a passive process: Health difficulties are conveyed to the doctor (or other professional), who then decides what must be done. The patient's responsibility is to follow the doctor's orders. The current generation of older people, in particular, are very respectful of a doctor's authority and may feel reluctant to clarify treatment plans or ask questions. An alternative approach to health care regards people as active consumers of health services. The consumer takes responsibility for clearly conveying the nature of his or her problem to the professional, for understanding the diagnostic assessment that is offered, for ascertaining what the professional intends to do about the problem, and for clarifying what the cost of treatment will be and the types of payment that will be accepted. Although the consumer/patient is usually not in a position to evaluate the technical competence of the professional from whom services are obtained, concerns about this can be addressed by requesting a second opinion from another professional. Too often people fail to find out basic facts about their medical care. For persons with mental health problems, it may be even more difficult to take an active consumer role. Family and friends can often be of considerable help in this regard.

For an individual who has located a mental health professional, the following questions may prove to be useful in becoming a better informed consumer of mental health services.

1. *What kind of mental health professional is the individual who is offering services?* Is he or she a psychiatrist, psychologist, psychiatric nurse, social worker, or other mental health service provider? What does his or her training permit him or her to do? Is he or she licensed? Does he or she have special expertise in provision of services to older adults? How was this expertise obtained? To what extent will confidentiality be maintained? The following is a brief description of different kinds of mental health professionals and the services they typically provide.

The Helping Professionals:
Who They Are—What They Do

Psychiatrists

A psychiatrist is a medical doctor who specializes in mental disorders, is licensed to practice medicine, and has completed three years of specialty training. A certified psychiatrist has, in addition, practiced for two years and passed the examinations of the American Board of Psychiatry and Neurology. Psychiatrists can evaluate and diagnose all types of mental disorders, carry out biomedical treatments and psychotherapy, and work with psychological problems associated with medical disorders. Of the mental health professionals, only psychiatrists can prescribe drugs and medical therapies. Child psychiatrists specialize in working with children; geriatric psychiatrists concentrate on helping the aged.

Psychologists

The field of psychology includes many specialties—clinical treatment, testing, community organization, industrial relations, laboratory research, and many more. Psychologists who conduct psychotherapy and work with individuals, groups, or families to resolve problems generally are called clinical psychologists, counseling psychologists, or school psychologists. They work in many settings—for example, mental health centers, hospitals and clinics, schools, employee assistance programs, and private practice. In most states, a licensed psychologist has completed a doctoral degree from a program with specialized training and experience requirements and has successfully completed a professional licensing examination.

Psychiatric Nurses

Psychiatric nursing is a specialized area of professional nursing practice that is concerned with prevention, treatment, and rehabilitation of mental health–related problems. These nurses are registered professional nurses who have advanced academic degrees at the master's degree level or above. They conduct individual, family, and group therapy and also work in mental health consultation, education, and administration.

Social Workers

Individual therapy, diagnosis, referral, consultation, and group therapy are some of the tasks that social workers are trained to perform. Psychiatric social workers have master's degrees in social work and have completed field-placement programs designed to train them in basic techniques in several areas, including therapy, community organization, administration, and consultation.

Psychotherapists

Psychotherapists are mental health professionals who treat patients. Some people who call themselves psychotherapists do not have adequate training. If you doubt the credentials of a therapist, check with [one of the organizations listed in Chapter 5, Directory of Organizations].

Mental Health Counselors

A clinical mental health counselor provides professional counseling services involving psychotherapy, human development, learning theory, and group dynamics to individuals, couples, and families. The promotion and enhancement of healthy, satisfying lifestyles are the goals of mental health counselors, whether the services are rendered in a mental health center, business, private practice, or other community agency. Clinical mental health counselors have earned at least a master's degree, and several years' clinical supervision is required before they are certified by the National Academy of Certified Clinical Mental Health Counselors.

Case Managers and Outreach Workers

These individuals assist severely or chronically mentally ill individuals, including the homeless mentally ill, to obtain the services they need to live in the community. Most chronically mentally ill persons need medical care, social services, and assistance from a variety of agencies, including those dealing with housing, Social Security, vocational rehabilitation, and mental health. Because such services are uncoordinated in many areas, case managers provide a critical function to monitor a person's needs and assure that appropriate agencies get involved. In many instances they also act as advocates for the client. Case managers can be nurses, social workers, or mental health workers and can be associated with mental health centers, psychosocial rehabilitation programs, and other agencies.

Reprinted from: National Institute of Mental Health. *A Consumer's Guide to Mental Health Services.* Revised, 1987. DHHS Publication No. (ADM) 87-214.

2. How much will evaluation and treatment cost? It is important to find out if the service provider accepts public or private health insurance and, if so, to what extent the insurance will cover anticipated costs of care. If services appear unaffordable, will the professional make alternative financial arrangements such as sliding-scale fees, whereby the individual pays according to need? If not, what other options does the professional suggest?

3. *How does the professional view the problem?* After evaluation, what is the diagnosis or tentative diagnosis? A clear, under-
standable explanation of the problem is deserved. If any of the
information is not understood, the service provider should be
contacted for further explanation.

4. *What is the plan for treating the problem?* What procedures
will likely be done? Will medication be prescribed? If so, what is
the medication and what are its possible side effects? If psychotherapy is recommended, what kind of psychotherapy? How
long will treatments likely last? Are there other treatment options? If so, why aren't they being considered at the present time?
Will it be necessary to work in conjunction with other health or
mental health professionals? If so, why and with whom?

5. *What is the likely outcome of treatment?* Although this can
rarely be stated with 100 percent certainty, the success rates of
many treatments have been researched. What does the service
provider know about the usual success rate? What does success
mean in this case: complete cure or alleviation of some symptoms? What is the service provider's own experience with the
success of the treatment that he or she is recommending?

When these or other questions need to be asked of the service
provider, it is sometimes helpful to write them down and bring
them to an appointment. Such a list becomes a sort of agenda
that will help guide a meeting with the health professional.

What if these and other questions remain unanswered or are
answered unsatisfactorily? It is reasonable to communicate this
concern and ask for further clarification of the issue. For example, some people are instructed to take medications at times that
are simply not convenient for them. If this is communicated to
the physician, he or she may develop a plan that more realistically accommodates the patient. If it should happen that the
patient and professional cannot come to agreement on how
treatment should proceed, it is often best to find another professional. It is important to note, however, that some people go
from one professional to another and are dissatisfied with what-
ever treatment plan is offered. This can be counterproductive
since it may delay receipt of needed treatment.

During the course of an agreed-upon treatment it is important for both professional and patient to periodically review goals and the progress that has been made toward achieving those goals. If goals are not being reached, it is important to discuss why this is happening. Perhaps other options need to be considered. It is often a matter of judgment about when, and if, the treatment plan should be changed. A mental health professional needs to follow a treatment plan long enough to make sure that it will work, if it is going to work. A good example is antidepressant medications. Most antidepressants take four to six weeks (and sometimes longer) to achieve their desired effect. Some physicians prematurely stop or change antidepressants because of frustration over the apparent lack of progress. This deprives the patient of the possible therapeutic benefit of a medication that will eventually work, creates the false impression that the patient is not responsive to the particular antidepressant, and possibly means that the patient will suffer with the symptoms of the mental disorder for longer than necessary.

On the other hand, patients have a right to discontinue treatments that have no benefit after they have tried the treatment for a reasonable amount of time. Professionals occasionally feel that they have exhausted all treatments that they feel capable of providing and may communicate this to the patient. Although the professional has a right to do this, he or she is also responsible for helping the patient to pursue other treatment options.

The critical issue is that there must be a free flow of information between the patient and the professional. Treatments are sometimes complex and success may not always be apparent. As long as the patient and the service provider honestly engage in a collaborative process, it is more likely that treatment goals will eventually be reached.

References for Part One

American Psychiatric Association. *Diagnostic and Statistical Manual of Mental Disorders, Third Edition, Revised.* Washington, DC: American Psychiatric Association, 1987.

Beckham, E. Edward, and William R. Leber, eds. *Handbook of Depression: Treatment, Assessment, and Research.* Homewood, IL: Dorsey Press, 1985.

Binstock, Robert H., and Ethel Shanas, eds. *Handbook of Aging and the Social Sciences.* 2d ed. New York: Van Nostrand, 1985.

Birren, James E., and K. Warner Schaie, eds. *Handbook of the Psychology of Aging.* 2d ed. New York: Van Nostrand, 1985.

Birren, James E., and R. Bruce Sloane, eds. *Handbook of Mental Health and Aging.* Englewood Cliffs, NJ: Prentice-Hall, 1980.

Blazer, Dan G. *Depression in Late Life.* St. Louis: C. V. Mosby Company, 1982.

Breslau, Lawrence D., and Marie R. Haug, eds. *Depression and Aging: Causes, Care, and Consequences.* New York: Springer, 1983.

Busse, Ewald W., and Dan G. Blazer, eds. *Geriatric Psychiatry.* Washington, DC: American Psychiatric Press, 1989.

Busse, Ewald W., and Dan G. Blazer, eds. *Handbook of Geriatric Psychiatry.* New York: Van Nostrand, 1980.

Butler, Robert N., and Myrna I. Lewis. *Aging and Mental Health: Positive Psychosocial and Biomedical Approaches.* 3d ed. Columbus, OH: Merrill, 1982.

Carstensen, Laura L., and Barry A. Edelstein, eds. *Handbook of Clinical Gerontology.* New York: Pergamon Press, 1987.

Hafner, H., G. Moschel, and N. Sartorius, eds. *Mental Health in the Elderly: A Review of the Present State of Research.* Berlin: Springer-Verlag, 1986.

Jenike, Michael A. *Handbook of Geriatric Psychopharmacology.* Littleton, MA: PSG Publishing Company, 1985.

Kermis, Marguerite D. *Mental Health in Later Life: The Adaptive Process.* Boston and Monterey, CA: Jones and Bartlett, 1986.

Lazarus, Lawrence W., ed. *Essentials of Geriatric Psychiatry: A Guide for Health Professionals.* New York: Springer, 1988.

Lewinsohn, Peter M., and Linda Teri, eds. *Clinical Geropsychology: New Directions in Assessment and Treatment.* New York: Pergamon Press, 1983.

Lurie, Elinore E., and James H. Swan, eds. *Serving the Mentally Ill Elderly: Problems and Perspectives.* Lexington, MA: Lexington Books, 1987.

Miller, Nancy E., and Gene D. Cohen, eds. *Schizophrenia and Aging: Schizophrenia, Paranoia, and Schizophreniform Disorders in Later Life.* New York: Guilford Press, 1987.

O'Conner, Kathleen, and Joyce Prothero, eds. *The Alzheimer Caregiver: Strategies for Support.* Seattle: University of Washington Press, 1986.

Poon, Leonard W., ed. *Aging in the 1980s.* Washington, DC: American Psychological Association, 1980.

Salzman, Carl. *Clinical Geriatric Psychopharmacology.* New York: McGraw-Hill, 1984.

Zarit, Steven H. *Aging and Mental Disorders: Psychological Approaches to Assessment and Treatment.* New York: Free Press, 1980.

Zarit, Steven H., Nancy K. Orr, and Judy M. Zarit. *The Hidden Victims of Alzheimer's Disease: Families under Stress.* New York: New York University Press, 1985.

Resources

Chapter 5

Directory of Organizations

National Resources

The following is a description of national organizations devoted to mental health and/or aging issues. The organizations include governmental agencies, professional groups, and self-help organizations. They have been selected on the basis of prominence in their respective fields and usefulness to persons seeking information about places to obtain mental health services or written materials on mental health and/or aging.

Alcoholics Anonymous (AA)
General Service Board of Alcoholics Anonymous, Inc.
P.O. Box 459
Grand Central Station
New York, NY 10163
(212) 686-1100

This is a worldwide organization of men and women who meet to try to attain and maintain sobriety. It is estimated that there are more than 1.5 million members in over 100 countries. AA is not directed by professionals and members of groups take an active hand in developing and coordinating local activities. A local AA group may usually be located in the phone book. AA produces a wide variety of printed and audiovisual materials that are available at minimal cost.

The Alzheimer's Association
(formerly The Alzheimer's Disease and Related Disorders Association)
Edward F. Truschke, President

70 East Lake Street
Chicago, IL 60601-5997
(800) 621-0379; in Illinois (800) 572-6037

> The Alzheimer's Association was founded in 1980 by families of people with dementia, physicians, and scientists. Its goals are to improve research, education, and public policy on dementing disorders. It sponsors more than 200 chapters that work locally to achieve its goals and to provide support groups and other services for families of people with dementia.
>
> SERVICES: Persons interested in information about or who wish to attend a local chapter meeting of the Alzheimer's Association may call the 24-hour toll-free numbers listed above or write to the association.
>
> PUBLICATIONS: A newsletter describing the organization's activities is published quarterly and often includes articles that discuss different issues in caring for a person with dementia. The association also publishes more than 30 brochures that would be of particular interest to dementia caregivers. A brief review of some of these brochures may be found in Chapter 6 in the section titled "Pamphlets." The association also publishes handbooks for people working with dementia patients and their families.

American Association for Geriatric Psychiatry
Alice Martinez, Executive Secretary
P.O. Box 376A
Greenbelt, MD 20770
(301) 220-0952

> The American Association for Geriatric Psychiatry (AAGP) was founded in 1978 for psychiatrists with an interest in mental health care for older adults. It carries out educational and informational activities including an annual meeting.
>
> SERVICES: The AAGP publishes a membership directory that lists name, address, phone number, professional background, and whether the member accepts patient referrals. Individuals interested in obtaining a copy of the AAGP membership directory (current as of 1987) may write to the above address.
>
> PUBLICATIONS: The organization produces a newsletter six times a year.

American Association of Retired Persons
Horace B. Deets, Executive Director
1909 K Street, NW
Washington, DC 20049
(202) 728-4300

> The American Association of Retired Persons (AARP) is a non-profit, nonpartisan organization founded in 1958 with a current membership of more than 28 million. It provides members (persons 50 years or older) with a wide range of services, lobbies for the interests of older individuals, has a gerontology resource center at its national headquarters, and sponsors many educational and service programs for older individuals. Of particular interest to older persons who take prescription medications is AARP's pharmacy service, through which members may obtain pharmaceuticals by mail (or in person at a few select locations) at reduced prices. Information about the pharmacy service may be obtained from: The AARP Pharmacy Service, 500 Montgomery Street, Alexandria, VA 22314; telephone (703) 684-0244.

> PUBLICATIONS: The AARP publishes *Modern Maturity,* a bimonthly magazine, and also produces a variety of publications, many of which are available free of charge. For a list of available publications write to the Office of Communications at the above Washington address. The AARP Pharmacy Service also distributes a series of 93 information leaflets on different prescription drugs. The leaflets—produced with the assistance of the U.S. Food and Drug Administration and experts in geriatric medicine and pharmacy—provide useful information on different types of drugs, how to properly take them, possible side effects, and information that the prescribing physician needs to know about the individual taking the medication.

The American Geriatrics Society
Linda Hiddemen Barondess, Vice President
770 Lexington Avenue, Suite 400
New York, NY 10021
(212) 308-1414

> The American Geriatrics Society (AGS) is a professional organization that was founded in 1942. The AGS is involved in educational (e.g., annual meeting, medical education, and accreditation), public policy, and publishing activities.

SERVICES: AGS does not provide referrals to individual physicians. It does publish a *Directory of Fellowship Programs in Geriatric Medicine* that lists places, names, phone numbers, and other information about training programs in geriatrics. These programs, which often deliver better clinical services than are usually found in the community, may be a good place to start in the search for medical and psychiatric services in a particular area. The directory is available (for $25 to nonmembers and $35 to institutions) by writing to AGS at the above address.

PUBLICATIONS: In addition to the above-mentioned directory, the AGS publishes the *Journal of the American Geriatrics Society* (a professional journal), the *Clinical Report on Aging* (a bimonthly tabloid on geriatric care), and two newsletters.

American Psychiatric Association
Melvin Sabshin, M.D., Medical Director
1400 K Street, NW
Washington, DC 20009
(202) 682-6220

The American Psychiatric Association (APA) is an organization of psychiatrists founded in 1844. The organization formulates mental health programs, compiles and distributes information about psychiatry, promotes psychiatric research and education, and maintains a library.

SERVICES: Individuals desiring information about psychiatric services in their area or a referral to a local psychiatrist may contact one of APA's local psychiatric societies. A list of the local societies is provided in this chapter in the section titled "State and Local Resources." The extent of assistance that can be provided varies among local societies.

PUBLICATIONS: The APA publishes two professional journals, *American Journal of Psychiatry* and *Hospital and Community Psychiatry*; a semimonthly newsletter, *Psychiatric News*; and a membership directory. For the general public, the APA publishes a series of 12 "Let's Talk Facts" brochures on select topics in mental health. Information about these brochures may be obtained by writing to: Facts About Series, APA Division of Public Affairs, at the above address. Several of these brochures are reviewed in Chapter 6 in the section titled "Pamphlets." The

American Psychiatric Press, the publishing arm of the APA, not only publishes its journals, but also produces a wide variety of books on mental health both for the professional and the general public. Several of these books are reviewed in Chapter 6 in the section titled "Books." Those interested in obtaining a list of current publications may write to the American Psychiatric Press at the above address.

American Psychological Association
Raymond D. Fowler, Chief Executive Officer
1200 17th Street, NW
Washington, DC 20036
(202) 955-7600

The American Psychological Association (APA) was founded in 1892. It is a scientific and professional association with a membership of almost 60,000. Its stated purpose is to "advance psychology as a science, as a profession, and as a means of promoting human welfare." It holds annual meetings, publishes a wide variety of journals, and works toward improving the quality of research, education, and services in psychology.

SERVICES: APA does not directly offer assistance in locating psychological services. Many of its local affiliates, however, may be able to provide more general guidance. Several affiliates have established referral systems to area psychologists. A list of APA affiliates may be found in this chapter in the section titled "State and Local Resources."

PUBLICATIONS: APA publishes a monthly newsletter, *APA Monitor,* and many professional journals, including *Psychology and Aging.* The organization also publishes books for professionals and maintains a computerized database of literature that would be of interest to psychologists and related disciplines.

American Society on Aging
Gloria Cavanaugh, Executive Director
833 Market Street, Suite 512
San Francisco, CA 94103
(415) 543-2617

The American Society on Aging (ASA) is a multidisciplinary group of administrators, service providers, educators, and others. It provides professional education on issues of current concern

in the field of gerontology, holds an annual meeting, and sponsors special projects.

SERVICES: ASA provides no direct services or referrals for the
general public.

PUBLICATIONS: ASA publishes a quarterly journal, *Generations,* each issue of which is devoted to a single topic regarding
aging, and a bimonthly newspaper, *The Aging Connection.* A list
of back issues of *Generations* is available (including issues on
caregivers, mental health, and alcohol and drugs) by writing to
ASA at the above address.

The Department of Veterans Affairs
Edward Derwinski, Department Secretary
810 Vermont Avenue, NW
Washington, DC 20420

The Department of Veterans Affairs (VA), previously known as
the Veterans Administration, provides a range of benefits to U.S.
veterans and their families. Perhaps the best known of VA
benefits are its hospitals and medical care services, which make
up one of the world's largest health care systems.

SERVICES: Eligibility for veteran benefits is a complex business
that takes into consideration the veteran's status, income, and a
host of other issues. People should contact their regional VA,
which can usually be found in the telephone book. Otherwise, an
individual may write to the VA to request the location of the
nearest office. In 1975 the VA established Geriatric Research,
Education, and Clinical Centers (GRECCs) that are involved in
research, education, and clinical services. At present there are 12
GRECCs, some of which specialize in the diagnosis of dementia
and depression. The GRECCs are listed in this chapter in the
section titled "State and Local Resources." Forty VA facilities
have specialized dementia inpatient services. Long-term care
(e.g., nursing homes) is available to some veterans. Contact the
local VA to obtain information on available services. However,
when seeking this information, be patient and persistent since the
VA is a large and often bureaucratic organization.

PUBLICATIONS: One publication of critical interest to those desiring VA-related medical services is the booklet *Federal Benefits for Veterans and Dependents.* This booklet outlines basic

eligibility criteria for different programs. It may be obtained from a local VA office.

Family Service America
Geneva B. Johnson, CEO and President
11700 West Lake Park Drive
Park Place
Milwaukee, WI 53224
(414) 359-1040

> Family Service America is the parent organization of 290 private, not-for-profit, independent agencies in the United States and Canada that help individuals and their families with different problems. The parent organization accredits and provides technical information to its local members.

> SERVICES: Although the activities of local Family Service America–affiliated organizations vary, all of them provide counseling to individuals and families to help them cope with personal problems. Some agencies have specialized services for the aged. An individual interested in finding a local Family Service America member may write a letter to the Information Center at the above address, accompanied by a stamped, self-addressed envelope. The organization prefers that telephone inquiries for this information are not made.

> PUBLICATIONS: Family Service America publishes the professional journal *Social Casework,* a newsletter, and books, videotapes, and audiotapes that would be of interest to the professional. A publication catalogue may be obtained by writing to the Publication Service at the above address.

Gerontological Society of America
John M. Corman, Executive Director
1411 K Street, NW, Suite 300
Washington, DC 20005
(202) 393-1411

> The Gerontological Society of America (GSA) is an interdisciplinary organization of professionals with interest in aging. It was founded in 1945 and promotes the scientific study of various aspects of aging, disseminates information about aging, and provides guidance to policymakers. GSA has more than 7,000

members and holds an annual scientific meeting. It is the most active and prominent gerontology organization in the United States.

SERVICES: GSA does not offer assistance to persons who are trying to find services for older adults.

PUBLICATIONS: GSA publishes *The Journals of Gerontology, Gerontologist,* and the monthly newsletter *Gerontology News.* The society also offers several publications for sale, including *Aging and Sensory Change: An Annotated Bibliography, Data Resources in Gerontology, Ties that Bind: The Interdependence of Generations, The Common Stake: The Interdependence of Generations* (a brief summary of the prior publication), and *Where Do We Come From? What Are We? Where Are We Going? An Annotated Bibliography of Aging and the Humanities.*

National Alliance for the Mentally Ill
Laurie M. Flynn, Executive Director
2101 Wilson Boulevard, Suite 302
Arlington, VA 22201
(703) 524-7600

The National Alliance for the Mentally Ill (NAMI) is a group founded in 1979 by families and friends of people with serious mental illnesses. It has grown considerably in the last ten years and currently has more than 80,000 members. It advocates the need for mental health services and research, educates the public about mental illness, and sponsors self-help groups for people with mental illness, their families, and their friends.

SERVICES: NAMI has chapters throughout the country that work to promote its goals on a local level and that sponsor support groups. Local NAMI affiliates will probably be a good resource for locating information about area mental health services. Interested persons should contact NAMI for the name and location of the closest NAMI affiliate.

PUBLICATIONS: NAMI publishes a newsletter, *The Advocate.* In addition, it publishes a variety of brochures, papers, and other materials, some of which are reviewed in Chapter 6 in the section titled "Pamphlets." NAMI sells a select group of books on mental illness at below retail cost.

National Association of Area Agencies on Aging
Raymond C. Mastalish, Executive Director
600 Maryland Avenue, SW
Washington, DC 20024
(202) 484-7520

The National Association of Area Agencies on Aging (NAAAA) is a private nonprofit organization that represents the interests of Area Agencies on Aging (AAAs) throughout the country. It provides information, technical assistance, and training to AAAs.

SERVICES: AAAs were developed in conjunction with the Older Americans Act (which mandated a broad range of services for older adults) and are designated by each state to address the needs and concerns of its citizens. AAA is a general term. The specific names of local AAAs vary, as do the geographical areas they cover (e.g., local, county, or multicounty). Although the services provided by AAAs vary by locale, one or several of the following may be provided: (1) access services such as assessment, case management, information and referral, outreach, and transportation; (2) community-based services such as meals, legal assistance, respite care, and employment services; (3) in-home services such as home health care, delivered meals, chore services, and supportive services for people caring for older individuals; and (4) other services such as casework and counseling and long-term care ombudsmen. The closest AAA will probably be a good place to try to get information about mental health services. If an individual finds it difficult to locate a local AAA, he or she may call the NAAAA, which will provide the name and number of the nearest agency.

PUBLICATIONS: The NAAAA publishes a newsletter and *The 1989–90 Directory of State and Area Agencies on Aging: A National Guide for Elder Care Information and Referral.* The directory includes names, addresses, and telephone numbers of AAAs and other agencies; descriptions of commonly provided elder care support services; and a section listing specialized publications and support groups for caregivers. It may be obtained for $30 by writing to the NAAAA at the above address.

National Association of Social Workers
Mark G. Battle, ACSW, Executive Director

7981 Eastern Avenue
Silver Spring, MD 29010
(301) 565-0333

> The National Association of Social Workers (NASW) is a professional organization for social workers. The NASW develops professional standards for social work, enforces ethical principles, engages in legislative and political action related to social service issues, educates the public, and provides a variety of services for its members.

> SERVICES: The NASW does not provide direct services to the general public. Nevertheless, the organization publishes a register of 20,000 names and telephone numbers of clinical social workers throughout the country. An individual interested in locating a clinical social worker may call the NASW national office at the telephone number above and ask for the Clinical Register Office. Local chapters of the NASW may also be able to provide some guidance in locating local resources. A list of local chapters of the NASW is provided in this chapter in the section titled "State and Local Resources."

> PUBLICATIONS: The NASW publishes the professional journals *Social Work, Health and Social Work, Social Work Research and Abstracts,* and *Social Work in Education*. It also produces a number of reference texts for social workers, a monthly newsletter, and a computer database of social work abstracts.

National Council of Community Mental Health Centers
Charles G. Ray, Executive Director
12300 Twinbrook Parkway, Suite 320
Rockville, MD 20852
(301) 984-6200

> The National Council of Community Mental Health Centers (NCCMHC) is an organization representing community mental health centers throughout the country. It lobbies Congress concerning mental health issues, provides information and supports to its members, and produces educational materials.

> SERVICES: Individuals who are unable to locate their local community mental health center may contact the council, which will provide this information.

PUBLICATIONS: The NCCMHC produces brochures, audio-visual materials, books, a professional journal (*Community Mental Health Journal*), and a newspaper. Of interest to those trying to locate mental health services, the organization produces the *National Registry of Community Mental Health Services*, which includes names, addresses, phone numbers, and other information about mental health services in the United States. It is available to nonmembers for $50. The registry and/or a list of publications/audiovisual materials may be obtained by writing to the NCCMHC at the above address. Of special note is the publication *Serving the Elderly: A Mental Health Resource Guide*, which is available to nonmembers for $45. This book is reviewed in Chapter 6 in the section titled "Books."

National Depressive and Manic Depressive Association
Lorraine Richter, Corresponding Secretary
Merchandise Mart, Box 3395
Chicago, IL 60654
(312) 939-2442

The National Depressive and Manic Depressive Association (NDMDA) was founded and is directed by people with mood disorders and their families. Working in consultation with the medical community, the NDMDA disseminates information on mood disorders, lobbies for improved research and services for people with mood disorders, and fosters the development of its more than 140 affiliates and support groups throughout the United States.

SERVICES: Persons interested in locating a local chapter of NDMDA or a support group should write to the above address. A current listing of chapters/support groups will be sent along with a packet of information about the organization. Local chapters may also be a good resource for those trying to locate mental health services in their area. The association asks that requests for information be made in writing due to a heavy volume of phone calls.

PUBLICATIONS: The association publishes a newsletter and sells, at a discount, books on mental health and audiocassettes of presentations at its national meetings.

The National Institute of Mental Health
Lewis L. Judd, M.D., Director
5600 Fishers Lane
Rockville, MD 20857
(301) 443-4513

> The National Institute of Mental Health (NIMH) is a governmental agency that conducts research; supports research, training, and certain "demonstration" mental health programs; assists other agencies in the development of mental health programs; and disseminates information. The Mental Disorders of the Aging Research Branch is the focus of NIMH's activities regarding mental health and aging.

> SERVICES: Persons interested in locating their local community mental health center may contact the Public Inquiries Office at the number listed above or write to this office at the address listed above.

> PUBLICATIONS: NIMH is a good source of information on a wide variety of mental health topics. The interested individual may request a list of current publications by writing to: Public Inquiries Branch, Room 15C-05, Office of Scientific Information, at the above address. Single copies of many publications are available free of charge. Several publications are reviewed in Chapter 6 in the section titled "Pamphlets."

National Institute on Aging
T. Franklin Williams, M.D., Executive Director
National Institutes of Health
Bethesda, Maryland 20892

National Institute on Aging Information Center
P.O. Box 8057
Gaithersburg, MD 20898-8057
(301) 495-3455

> The National Institute on Aging (NIA) was established by Congress in 1974 and charged with responsibility for conducting and supporting research and training on various aspects of aging.

> SERVICES: The NIA currently sponsors 12 Alzheimer's Disease Research Centers (ADRCs) that research various aspects of Alzheimer's disease. Since some ADRCs have treatment protocols

or services, those who live in the geographical locale of an ADRC may be interested in getting further information about its activities. Persons interested in the work of individual ADRCs may contact the NIA Information Center, whose address is above.

PUBLICATIONS: The NIA produces a variety of publications on aging both for the professional and for the general public. These include information packets about the NIA, Alzheimer's disease, research and grant opportunities, health education, and disease prevention; technical reports and research summaries; and *Age Pages* — brief health summaries for the general public on various topics. Some of these summaries are available in Spanish or in Chinese languages. Some of the publications available from NIA are summarized in Chapter 6 in the section titled "Pamphlets."

National Mental Health Association
Preston Garrison, Executive Director
1021 Prince Street
Alexandria, VA 22314-2971
(703) 684-7722

The National Mental Health Association is the nation's oldest and largest citizens' voluntary mental health organization. It is an educational and social advocacy organization that promotes mental health awareness, education, and prevention of mental illness. Local mental health associations provide information to individuals and community groups, support and assistance to persons with mental illness and their families, and education about mental illness to school systems, local governments, and other organizations.

SERVICES: The National Mental Health Association may be contacted if individuals are seeking the name of the closest mental health association in their area. Some mental health associations provide referrals to mental health resources in their communities. State mental health associations exist throughout most parts of the country and they also may be contacted for information. A listing of state mental health associations is included in this chapter in the section titled "State and Local Resources."

PUBLICATIONS: The National Mental Health Association publishes a variety of brochures on mental health. An individual may write or phone the association for a listing of available brochures.

Some brochures are described in Chapter 6 in the section titled "Pamphlets."

The National Mental Health Consumers Self-Help Clearinghouse
Joseph Rogers, Executive Director
311 South Juniper Street, Suite 902
Philadelphia, PA 19107
(215) 735-6367

The clearinghouse, conducted in collaboration with the Mental Health Association of Southeastern Pennsylvania and Project SHARE, provides information and referral services to individuals and groups throughout the country, offers onsite consultation and training for groups concerned with mental health issues, awards some funding for technical assistance projects, and maintains a library of materials.

SERVICES: Individuals seeking information about self-help groups for consumers of mental health services may phone or write the organization. Self-help groups may be of assistance in helping the individual find local mental health resources.

PUBLICATIONS: The clearinghouse has a library of materials on more than 100 topics, copies of which are available for a slight charge to cover photocopying and postage.

State and Local Resources

The following is a group of organizations that have affiliates or chapters that may be useful sources of information on local resources. Also see the previous section in this chapter, "National Resources," for a description of most of the parent organizations of these groups.

Alzheimer's Disease Research Centers

The National Institute on Aging funds 12 Alzheimer's Disease Research Centers that are currently investigating the causes and possible treatments for dementia. Some of them offer services in connection with research studies that may be of interest to families of persons with dementia.

California
University of California, San Diego
Department of Neurosciences (M-024)
UCSD School of Medicine
La Jolla, CA 92093
(619) 534-4606
Director: Robert Katzman, M.D.

University of Southern California
Andrus Gerontology Center
University Park, MC-0191
Los Angeles, CA 90089-0191
(213) 743-5168
Director: Caleb E. Finch, Ph.D.

Kentucky
University of Kentucky
Sanders-Brown Research Center on
  Aging
Lexington, KY 40536-0230
(606) 233-6040
Director: William R. Markesbery, M.D.

Maryland
The Johns Hopkins Medical
  Institutions
Department of Pathology
The Johns Hopkins Hospital
600 North Wolfe Street
Baltimore, MD 21205
(301) 955-5632
Director: Donald L. Price, M.D.

Massachusetts
Harvard Medical School
Massachusetts General Hospital
Department of Neurology
ACC 730
Fruit Street
Boston, MA 02114
(617) 726-1728
Director: John H. Growdon, M.D.

Missouri
Washington University
School of Medicine
Alzheimer's Disease Research Center
16304 Barnes Hospital Plaza
St. Louis, MO 63110
(314) 367-3122
Director: Leonard Berg, M.D.

New York
Mt. Sinai School of Medicine
Bronx VA Medical
Department of Psychiatry
One Gustave L. Levy Place
New York, NY 10029-6571
(212) 241-6623
Director: Kenneth D. Davis, M.D.

North Carolina
Duke University
Division of Neurology
Memory Disorders Clinic
Duke University Medical Center
725 Broad Street
Durham, NC 27705
(919) 684-6274
Director: Allen D. Roses, M.D.

Ohio
Case Western Reserve University
Alzheimer Center
University Hospitals of Cleveland
2074 Abington Road
Cleveland, OH 44106
(216) 844-7360
Director: Peter Whitehouse, M.D.

Pennsylvania
University of Pittsburgh
Alzheimer's Disease Research Program
Iroquois Building, Suite 400
3600 Forbes Avenue
Pittsburgh, PA 15213
(412) 647-2160
Director: F. Jacob Huff, M.D.

Texas
University of Texas
Southwestern Medical Center
Department of Neurology
5323 Harry Hines Boulevard
Dallas, TX 75235-9036
Director: Roger N. Rosenberg, M.D.

Washington
University of Washington
Department of Pathology, SM-30
Seattle, WA 98185
(206) 543-5088
Director: George M. Martin, M.D.

American Psychiatric Association: Local Psychiatric Societies

Alabama
Alabama Psychiatric Society
P.O. Box 66311
Birmingham, AL 35210
(205) 933-7724

Alaska
Alaska District Branch of the American
  Psychiatric Association
4001 Dale Street, No. 101
Anchorage, AK 99508
(907) 561-1361

Arizona
Arizona Psychiatric Society
Desert Vista Hospital
570 West Brown Road
Mesa, AZ 85201
(602) 898-3314

Arkansas
Arkansas Psychiatric Society
UAMS Department of Psychiatry
4301 West Markham, Slot 554
Little Rock, AR 72205
(501) 661-5587

California
Central California Psychiatric Society
748 Plum Lane
Davis, CA 95616
(916) 753-2401

Northern California Psychiatric Society
1631 Ocean Avenue
San Francisco, CA 94112
(415) 334-2418

Orange County Psychiatric Society
300 South Flower Street, P.O. Box 1297
Orange, CA 92668
(714) 978-3016

San Diego Society of Psychiatric
  Physicians
7159 Navajo Road, No. 120
San Diego, CA 92119
(619) 582-3221

Southern California Psychiatric Society
2601 Ocean Park Boulevard, Suite 314
Santa Monica, CA 90405
(213) 450-4610

Colorado
Colorado Psychiatric Society
5991 South Bellaire Way
Littleton, CO 80121
(303) 220-9565

Connecticut
Connecticut Psychiatric Society
One Regency Drive, P.O. Box 30
Bloomfield, CT 06002
(203) 243-3977

Delaware
Delaware Psychiatric Association
Academy of Medicine Building
1925 Lovering Avenue
Wilmington, DE 19806
(302) 428-2961

District of Columbia
Washington Psychiatric Society
1400 K Street, NW
Washington, DC 20005
(202) 682-6192

Florida
Florida Psychiatric Society
P.O. Box 10002
Tallahassee, FL 32302
(904) 222-8404

South Florida Psychiatric Society, Inc.
P.O. Box 331266
Miami, FL 33133
(305) 854-6802

Georgia
Georgia Psychiatric Association
938 Peachtree Street, NE
Atlanta, GA 30309
(404) 876-7535

Hawaii
Hawaii Psychiatric Society
3879 Lurline Drive
Honolulu, HI 96816
(808) 732-3304

Idaho
Idaho District Branch of the American
   Psychiatric Association
0309 Second Street
Lewiston, ID 83501
(208) 743-8095

Illinois
Illinois Psychiatric Society
20 North Michigan Avenue, Suite 700
Chicago, IL 60602
(312) 263-7391

Indiana
Indiana Psychiatric Society
5331 Glen Stewart Way
Indianapolis, IN 46254
(317) 293-4770

Northern Indiana Psychiatric Society
701 Wall Street
Valparaiso, IN 46383
(219) 464-8541

Iowa
Iowa Psychiatric Society
1001 Grand Avenue
West Des Moines, IA 50265
(515) 223-1401

Kansas
Kansas Psychiatric Society
1259 Pembroke Lane
Topeka, KS 66604
(913) 232-5985

Kentucky
Kentucky Psychiatric Association
P.O. Box 198
Frankfort, KY 40602
(502) 695-4843

Louisiana
Louisiana Psychiatric Association
P.O. Box 15765
New Orleans, LA 70175
(504) 891-1030

Maine
Maine Psychiatric Association
RFD No. 1, P.O. Box 1620
North Whitefield, ME 04353
(207) 549-5786

Maryland
Maryland Psychiatric Society, Inc.
1204 Maryland Avenue
Baltimore, MD 21201
(301) 625-0232

Massachusetts
Massachusetts Psychiatric Society
One Washington Street, Suite 210
Wellesley, MA 02181
(617) 237-8100

Michigan
Michigan Psychiatric Society
21700 Northwestern Highway,
  Suite 1150
Southfield, MI 48075
(313) 552-8666

Minnesota
Minnesota Psychiatric Society
1770 Colvin Avenue
St. Paul, MN 55116
(612) 698-1971

Mississippi
Mississippi Psychiatric Association
Mississippi State Medical Association
735 Riverside Drive, P.O. Box 5229
Jackson, MS 39216
(601) 354-5433

Missouri
Central Missouri Psychiatric Society
2401 Bernadette, Suite 204
Columbia, MO 65203-4672
(314) 445-6444

Eastern Missouri Psychiatric Society
3839 Lindell Boulevard
St. Louis, MO 63108
(314) 371-5226

Western Missouri District Branch of the
  American Psychiatric Association
3036 Gillham Road
Kansas City, MO 64108
(816) 531-8432

Montana
Montana Psychiatric Association
College Professional Building
2520 17th Street, West
Billings, MT 59102
(406) 259-1425

Nebraska
Nebraska Psychiatric Society
Immanuel Hospital
6901 North 72nd Street
Omaha, NE 68122
(402) 572-2907

Nevada
Nevada Association of Psychiatric
  Physicians
The Montevista Center
5900 West Rochelle Avenue
Las Vegas, NV 89103
(702) 364-1111 ext. 103

New Hampshire
New Hampshire Psychiatric Society
76 South State Street, P.O. Box 1382
Concord, NH 03302
(603) 228-1231

New Jersey
New Jersey Psychiatric Association
803 Partridge Drive
Bridgewater, NJ 08807
(201) 685-0650

New Mexico
Psychiatric Medical Association of New
  Mexico
P.O. Box 26666
Albuquerque, NM 87125
(505) 841-3511

New York
Bronx District Branch of the American
  Psychiatric Association
78 Woodcrest Avenue
White Plains, NY 10604
(914) 946-3105

Brooklyn Psychiatric Society, Inc.
Four Chimney Court
Brookhaven, NY 11719
(516) 286-8907

Central New York District Branch of the
American Psychiatric Association
122 Orvilton Drive
DeWitt, NY 13214
(315) 446-0944

Genessee Valley Psychiatric Association
16 North Goodman Street
Rochester, NY 14607
(716) 461-2155

Mid-Hudson District Branch of the
American Psychiatric Association
141 Van Wagner Road
Poughkeepsie, NY 12603
(914) 452-5894

Nassau Psychiatric Society
400 Sunrise Highway
Amityville, NY 11701
(516) 691-8080

New York County District Branch of the
American Psychiatric Association
150 East 58th Street, 16th Floor
New York, NY 10022
(212) 421-4732/33/34

New York State Capital District Branch
of the American Psychiatric
Association
P.O. Box 5
New Baltimore, NY 12121
(518) 756-8149

Northern New York District Branch of
the American Psychiatric Association
1400 Noyes Street
Utica, NY 13502
(315) 797-6800

Queens County District Branch of the
American Psychiatric Association
47-04 159th Street
Flushing, NY 11358
(718) 461-8413

Suffolk County District Branch of the
American Psychiatric Association
3 Old Landers Court
Smithtown, NY 11787
(516) 265-5134

West Hudson District Branch of the
American Psychiatric Association
36 College Avenue
Nanuet, NY 10954
(914) 358-1687

Westchester County District Branch of
the American Psychiatric Association
Erie County Medical Center
78 Woodcrest Avenue
White Plains, NY 10604
(914) 946-9008

Western New York Psychiatric Society
462 Grider Street
Buffalo, NY 14215
(716) 898-3251

North Carolina
North Carolina Psychiatric Association
4917 Waters Edge Drive, Suite 250
Raleigh, NC 27606
(919) 859-3370

North Dakota
North Dakota District Branch of the
American Psychiatric Association
700 First Avenue South
Fargo, ND 58103
(701) 235-5354

Ohio
Ohio Psychiatric Association
c/o Ohio State Medical Association
600 South High Street
Columbus, OH 43215
(614) 228-6971

Oklahoma
Oklahoma Psychiatric Association
P.O. Box 1328
Norman, OK 73070
(405) 321-4514

Oregon
Oregon Psychiatric Association
1700 S.W. Columbia
Portland, OR 97201
(503) 224-6364

Pennsylvania
Pennsylvania Psychiatric Society
20 Erford Road
Lemoyne, PA 17043
(717) 763-7151

Puerto Rico
Puerto Rico Psychiatric Society
Mepsi Center
Call Box 6089
Bayamon, PR 00621-6089
(809) 793-3030

Rhode Island
Rhode Island Psychiatric Society
204 Taber Avenue
Providence, RI 02906
(401) 246-1195

South Carolina
South Carolina Psychiatric Association
1214 Henderson Street
Columbia, SC 29201
(803) 765-1498

South Dakota
South Dakota Psychiatric Association
800 East 21st Street
Sioux Falls, SD 57101
(605) 339-6785

Tennessee
Tennessee Psychiatric Association
112 Louise Avenue
Nashville, TN 37203
(615) 478-0605

Texas
Texas Society of Psychiatric Physicians
400 West 15th Street, Suite 1018
Austin, TX 78701
(512) 478-0605

Utah
Utah Psychiatric Association
540 East 500 South
Salt Lake City, UT 84108
(801) 355-7477

Vermont
Vermont Psychiatric Association
c/o Thomas Chittenden Health Center
Williston, VT 05495
(802) 879-0242

Virginia
Psychiatric Society of Virginia
209 Culpepper Road
Richmond, VA 23229
(804) 282-1231

Washington
Washington State Psychiatric
  Association
11626 13th Street S.W.
Seattle, WA 98146
(206) 248-3868

West Virginia
West Virginia Psychiatric Association
P.O. Box 630, West Virginia Medical
  Center
Department of Behavioral
  Medicine/Psychiatry
Morgantown, WV 26506
(304) 293-2411

Wisconsin
Wisconsin Psychiatric Association
P.O. Box 1109
Madison, WI 53701
(608) 257-6781

Wyoming
Wyoming Psychiatric Society
P.O. Box 1005
Cheyenne, WY 82001
(307) 634-9653

Canada

Ontario District Branch of the American
   Psychiatric Association
600 University Avenue, 9N, Room 942
Toronto, Ontario, Canada M5G 1X5
(416) 589-4569

Quebec & Eastern Canada District
   Branch of the American Psychiatric
   Association
Hospital Suite Therese
1705 George Avenue
Shawinegan, Quebec, Canada G9N 2N1
(819) 537-9351

Western Canada District Branch of the
   American Psychiatric Association
Vancouver General Hospital
715 West 12th Avenue
Vancouver, British Columbia, Canada
   V5Z 1M9
(604) 875-4515

American Psychological Association:
Affiliated State Psychological Associations

Alabama Psychological Association
P.O. Box 97
Montgomery, AL 36101-0097
(205) 262-8245

Alaska Psychological Association
Executive Officer
3211 Providence Drive
Anchorage, AK 99508
(907) 786-1718

Arizona Psychological Association
3602 East Campbell
Phoenix, AZ 85108
(602) 955-7703

Arkansas Psychological Association
6900 Incas Drive
North Little Rock, AR 72116
(501) 8344-2856

California State Psychological
   Association
1010 Eleventh Street, Suite 202
Sacramento, CA 95814
(916) 442-0271
Referral service to psychologists
   available.

Colorado Psychological Association
720 South Colorado Boulevard,
   Suite 465
Denver, CO 80222
(303) 692-9303
Referral service to psychologists
   available.

Connecticut Psychological Association
60 Washington Street, Suite 203
Hartford, CT 06106
(203) 549-2445
Referral service to psychologists
   available.

Delaware Psychological Association
P.O. Box 718
Claymont, DE 19703
(302) 475-1574

District of Columbia Psychological
   Association
1010 Hamlin Street, NE
Washington, DC 20017
(202) 232-6713
Referral service to psychologists
   available.

Florida Psychological Association
1377 East Tennessee Street
Tallahassee, FL 32308
(904) 656-2222

Georgia Psychological Association
1170 14th Place
Atlanta, GA 30309
(404) 874-5219

Hawaii Psychological Association
P.O. Box 10465
Honolulu, HI 96816
(808) 377-5992
Referral service to psychologists
   available.

Idaho Psychological Association
P.O. Box 8585
Boise, ID 83707
(208) 345-3072

Illinois Psychological Association
203 North Wabash, No. 2106
Chicago, IL 60601
(312) 372-7610

Indiana Psychological Association
310 North Alabama, Suite A
Indianapolis, IN 46204
(317) 636-6059

Iowa Psychological Association
P.O. Box 320
Knoxville, IA 50138
(515) 828-5035

Kansas Psychological Association
400 S.W. Croix
Topeka, KS 66611
(913) 267-7435

Kentucky Psychological Association
Keller Child Psychiatry Research Center
University of Louisville
Health Science Center
Louisville, KY 40292
(502) 588-5326

Louisiana Psychological Association
P.O. Box 66924
Baton Rouge, LA 70896
(504) 344-8839

Maine Psychological Association
71 Sewall Street
Augusta, ME 04330
(207) 622-1777

Maryland Psychological Association
1000 Century Plaza, No. 124
Columbia, MD 21044
(301) 992-4258

Massachusetts Psychological
   Association
14 Beacon Street, No. 704
Boston, MA 02108
(617) 523-6320

Michigan Psychological Association
29446 Ravine Drive
Livonia, MI 48152
(313) 525-0460

Minnesota Psychological Association
525 Park Street, Suite 310
St. Paul, MN 55103
(612) 293-1873
Referral service to psychologists available.

Mississippi Psychological Association
Highland Village, Suite 204
2500 I-55 North
Jackson, MS 39211-5931
(601) 362-9852

Missouri Psychological Association
1311 Lindbergh Plaza Center
St. Louis, MO 63132
(314) 993-3707

Montana Psychological Association
913 26th Street, S.W.
Great Falls, MT 59404
(406) 761-4226

Nebraska Psychological Association
11315 Chicago Circle
Omaha, NE 68154
(402) 333-0620
Referral service to psychologists
available.

Nevada Psychological Association
432 Court Street, Suite 202
Reno, NV 80500
(702) 322-5980

New Hampshire Psychological
Organization
Professional Services
2¹/2 Beacon Street, P.O. Box 1215
Concord, NH 03302
(603) 224-1816

New Jersey Psychological Association
349 East Northfield Road, Suite 211
Livingston, NJ 07039
(201) 535-9888
Referral service to psychologists
available.

New Mexico Psychological Association
P.O. Box 4068
Albuquerque, NM 87196
(505) 260-5560

New York State Psychological
Association
40 Central Avenue
Albany, NY 12206-3002
(518) 426-8911

North Carolina Psychological
Association
P.O. Box 33731
Raleigh, NC 27636-3731
(919) 781-4843

North Dakota Psychological Association
North Central Human Service Center
400 22nd Avenue, N.W.
Minot, ND 58701
(701) 852-1251

Ohio Psychological Association
400 East Town Street, Suite 020
Columbus, OH 43215
(614) 224-0034
Referral service to psychologists
available.

Oklahoma Psychological Association
116 Dean A. McGee Avenue
Oklahoma City, OK 73102
(405) 236-8547

Oregon Psychological Association
1750 Skyline Boulevard, Suite 12
Portland, OR 97221
(503) 292-4914

Pennsylvania Psychological Association
416 Forster Street
Harrisburg, PA 17102-1714
(717) 232-3817

Asociacion de Psicologos de Puerto Rico
Apartado 3435-Oficina General de
  Correo
San Juan, PR 00936
(809) 751-7100

Rhode Island Psychological Association
Independence Square
500 Prospect Street
Pawtucket, RI 02860
(401) 728-5570

South Carolina Psychological
  Association
P.O. Box 5207
Columbia, SC 29250
(803) 771-6050
Referral service to psychologists
  available.

South Dakota Psychological Association
P.O. Box 1037
Pierre, SD 57501
(605) 224-1034

Tennessee Psychological Association
530 Church Street, Suite 501
Nashville, TN 37219
(615) 321-5002

Texas Psychological Association
6633 East Highway 290, Suite 305
Austin, TX 78723
(512) 454-2449

Utah Psychological Association
P.O. Box 510960
Salt Lake City, UT 84151
(801) 364-9103

Vermont Psychological Association
P.O. Box 1017
Montpelier, VT 05602
(802) 229-5447

Virginia Psychological Association
109 Amherst Street
Winchester, VA 22601
(703) 667-5544

Washington State Psychological
  Association
13500 Lake City Way Northeast, No.
  208
Seattle, WA 98125
(206) 363-9772
Referral service to psychologists
  available.

West Virginia Psychological Association
P.O. Box 667
Charleston, WV 25323
(304) 345-2716

Wisconsin Psychological Association
121 South Hancock Street
Madison, WI 53703
(608) 251-1450

Wyoming Psychological Association
P.O. Box 1191
Laramie, WY 82070
(307) 745-3846

Canada

Ontario Psychological Association
730 Yonge Street, Suite 221
Toronto, Ontario M4Y 2B7
(416) 961-5552
Referral service to psychologists
  available.

Corporation Professionnelle des
  Psychologues du Quebec (CPPQ)
1100 Rue Beaumont
Ville Mont-Royal, Quebec H3P 3E5
(514) 738-1881
Referral service to psychologists
  available.

Department of Veterans Affairs: Geriatric Research, Education, and Clinical Centers (GRECCs)

Arkansas
Little Rock GRECC
Director: D. Lipschitz, M.D., Ph.D.
VA Medical Center
Little Rock, AR 72206
(501) 661-1202 ext. 2811

California
Palo Alto GRECC
Director: G. M. Reaven, M.D.
VA Medical Center
Palo Alto, CA 94304
(415) 858-3933

Sepulveda GRECC
Director: Information unavailable
VA Medical Center
Sepulveda, CA 91343
(818) 891-7711 ext. 2484

West Los Angeles GRECC
Director: T. Makinodan, Ph.D.
VA Medical Center
Los Angeles, CA 90073
(213) 824-4301

Florida
Gainesville GRECC
Director: D. Lowenthal, M.D.
VA Medical Center
Gainesville, FL 32602
(904) 374-6077

Massachusetts
Boston GRECC
Bedford Division
Director: R. E. Fine, Ph.D.
VA Medical Center
Bedford, MA 01730
(617) 275-7500 ext. 0631

Boston GRECC
Brockton/West Roxbury Division
Director: K. Minaker, M.D.
VA Medical Center
West Roxbury, MA 02132
(617) 323-7700 ext. 5990

Michigan
Ann Arbor GRECC
Director: Jeffrey Halter, M.D.
VA Medical Center
Ann Arbor, MI 48105
(313) 769-7100 ext. 7493

Minnesota
Minneapolis GRECC
Director: G. J. Maletta, M.D., Ph.D.
VA Medical Center
Minneapolis, MN 55417
(612) 725-2051 ext. 6313

Missouri
St. Louis GRECC
Director: J. E. Morley, M.D.
VA Medical Center
St. Louis, MO 63125
(314) 894-6510

North Carolina
Durham GRECC
Director: H. J. Cohen, M.D.
VA Medical Center
Durham, NC 27705
(919) 286-6932 ext. 6492

Texas
San Antonio GRECC
Director: Michael Katz, M.D.
VA Medical Center
San Antonio, TX 78284
(512) 694-5197

Washington
Seattle GRECC
American Lake Division
Director: R. C. Veith, M.D.
VA Medical Center
Tacoma, WA 98493
(206) 582-8440 ext. 6930

Seattle GRECC
Seattle Division
Director: R. C. Veith, M.D.
VA Medical Center
Seattle, WA 91808
(206) 764-2308

Geriatric Psychiatry Fellowship Programs

The following is a list of training programs for psychiatrists who plan to specialize in geriatrics. Sometimes these programs are conducted in conjunction with innovative services for older adults with mental health problems. Unfortunately, no central listing of all geriatric psychiatry fellowship programs exists, so these are gleaned from a variety of sources. The directors of programs sometimes change and occasionally fellowship programs are discontinued. Contacting one of the programs below will, nevertheless, offer an important first step in locating local mental health resources for older adults. The American Association for Geriatric Psychiatry (refer to the section in this chapter titled "National Resources") maintains a list of some geriatric psychiatry fellowship programs that is intermittently updated.

Alabama
University of Alabama at Birmingham
David Folks, M.D.
University Station
Birmingham, AL 35294

California
Stanford University School of Medicine
Jerome A. Yesavage, M.D.
Department of Psychiatry TD114
Stanford University School of Medicine
Stanford, CA 94305

University of California, Irvine
Thomas Cesario, M.D.
101 The City Drive, Building 53
Orange, CA 92668

University of California, Los Angeles,
  U.C.L.A. School of Medicine
James Spar, M.D.
UCLA Neuropsychiatric Institute
760 Westwood Plaza
Los Angeles, CA 90024

University of California, San Diego,
  School of Medicine
Dilip V. Jeste, M.D.
V-116A, San Diego VAMC
3350 La Jolla Village Drive
San Diego, CA 92161

University of Southern California School
of Medicine
Lon S. Schneider, M.D.
Department of Psychiatry
University of Southern California School
of Medicine
2025 Zonal Avenue
Los Angeles, CA 90033

Connecticut
Yale University
Alan Segal, M.D.
20 York Street
New Haven, CT 06504
(203) 785-4628

District of Columbia
Georgetown University School of
Medicine
Nathan Billig, M.D.
Georgetown University School of
Medicine
5410 Connecticut Avenue, NW
Washington, DC 20016

Florida
University of South Florida College of
Medicine
Eugene M. Dagon, M.D.
Department of Psychiatry, James Haley
VAMC
13000 Bruce Down Boulevard
Tampa, FL 33612

Illinois
Northwestern University Medical
School
Sanford Finkel, M.D.
Geriatric Psychiatry Services
259 East Erie Street, Suite 446
Chicago, IL 60611

Rush Medical College of Rush University
Lawrence W. Lazarus, M.D.
Johnston R. Bowman Center for the
Elderly
Rush Medical College of Rush University
1725 West Harrison Street
Chicago, IL 60612

Indiana
Indiana University School of Medicine
Hugh Hendrie, M.D.
534 Clinical Drive, Cottage, Room 110
Indianapolis, IN 46223

Louisiana
Louisiana State University School of
Medicine
Kenneth Sakauye, M.D.
Louisiana State University Medical Center
New Orleans, LA 70112

Maryland
Johns Hopkins University School of
Medicine
Peter V. Rabins, M.D.
Meyer 279, 600 North Wolfe Street
Baltimore, MD 21205

University of Maryland School of
Medicine
Paul Ruskin, M.D.
Baltimore VA Medical Center
3900 Loch Raven Boulevard
Baltimore, MD 21218

Massachusetts
Harvard Medical School–McLean
Hospital
Benjamin Liptzin, M.D.
115 Mill Street
Belmont, MA 02178

Massachusetts Mental Health Center
Bennett Gurian, M.D.
74 Fenwood Road
Boston, MA 02115

Minnesota
University of Minnesota Medical
    School–Minneapolis
Gabe Maletta, Ph.D., M.D.
54th and 48th Avenue South
Minneapolis, MN 55417

Missouri
St. Louis University School of Medicine
George T. Grossberg, M.D.
Division of Geriatric Psychiatry
St. Louis University Medical Center,
    Room 207
1221 South Grand Boulevard
St. Louis, MO 63104

New York
Albert Einstein College of Medicine
Gary Kennedy, M.D.
111 East 210th Street
Bronx, NY 10467

Columbia University Faculty of Medicine
John Toner, M.D.
Center for Geriatrics and Gerontology
100 Haven Avenue, Tower 3-30F
New York, NY 10032

Cornell University Medical College
Charles A. Shamoian, M.D., Ph.D.
New York Hospital–Cornell Medical
    Center, Westchester Division
21 Bloomingdale Road
White Plains, NY 10605

Hillside Hospital, A Division of Long
    Island Jewish Medical Center
Blaine Greenwald, M.D.
Hillside Hospital, Research Building
P.O. Box 38
Glen Oaks, NY 11004

New York University
Jeffrey R. Foster, M.D.
Department of Psychiatry
550 First Avenue
New York, NY 10016

State University of New York Health
    Science Center at Brooklyn
Carl Cohen, M.D.
Box 1203
450 Clarkson Avenue
Brooklyn, NY 11203

University of Rochester School of
    Medicine and Dentistry
David D. Bonacci, M.D.
P.O. Box Psychiatry
30-0 Crittenden Boulevard
Rochester, NY 14642

North Carolina
Bowman Gray College of Medicine
Burton Reifler, M.D.
Department of Psychiatry & Behavioral
    Medicine
Bowman Gray College of Medicine
Winston-Salem, NC 27103

Duke University
Dan Blazer, M.D.
Professor of Psychiatry
P.O. Box 3215
Duke University Medical Center
Durham, NC 27710

Ohio
University of Cincinnati College of
    Medicine
David Bienenfeld, M.D.
Department of Psychiatry, ML 559
University of Cincinnati College of
    Medicine
Cincinnati, OH 45267

Pennsylvania
Medical College of Pennsylvania
Ira R. Katz, M.D.
EPPI Division
Department of Psychiatry
3200 Henry Avenue
Philadelphia, PA 19129

University of Pennsylvania School of Medicine
G. L. Gottlieb, M.D.
HUP 3 Piersol/4283
3400 Spruce Street
Philadelphia, PA 19104

University of Pittsburgh School of Medicine
John P. Nelson, M.D.
3811 O'Hara Street
Pittsburgh, PA 15213

Washington
University of Washington School
  of Medicine
Murray Raskind, M.D.
GRECC (182-B)
Seattle VA Medical Center
1550 Columbia Way South
Seattle, WA 98108

Model Community Mental Health Programs for Older Adults

In 1988 the National Council of Community Mental Health Centers identified and surveyed 23 community programs that were providing innovative programming to meet the mental health needs of older adults. The following list of innovative programs is reproduced, with permission, from the National Council of Community Mental Health Centers' publication *Surveying the Elderly: A Mental Health Resource Guide*. Information on purchasing this publication may be found in the listing for the National Council of Community Mental Health Centers in the "National Resources" section of this chapter.

California
Didi Hirsch Community Mental Health
  Center
4760 South Sepulveda Boulevard
Culver City, CA 90230
(213) 390-6612

Colorado
Center for Mental Health
P.O. Box 1208
Montrose, CO 81401
(303) 249-0711

Florida
ACT Corporation
Hugh West Gerontology Center
1251 North Stone Street
DeLand, FL 32720
(904) 734-0440

Life Management Center of Northwest
  Florida
525 East 15th Street
Panama City, FL 32401
(904) 769-9481

Manatee Glens Corporation
P.O. Box 9478
Brandenton, FL 34206
(813) 758-9515

Iowa
Abbe Center
520 11th Street, N.W.
Cedar Rapids, IA 52405
(319) 398-3562

Kansas
Johnson County Mental Health Center
6000 Lamar Avenue
Mission, KS 66202
(913) 384-1100

Kentucky
Northern Kentucky Comprehensive
  Care Center
722 Scott Street
Covington, KY 41011
(606) 431-3052

Seven Counties Services, Inc.
101 West Muhammed Ali Boulevard
Louisville, KY 40202
(502) 585-5947

Maine
Tri-County Mental Health Services
465 Main Street
Lewiston, ME 04240
(207) 783-4676

Michigan
Neighborhood Services Organization
2111 Woodward, 3rd Floor
Detroit, MI 48201
(313) 961-7990

Van Buren County Mental Health
  Center
P.O. Box 249
Paw Paw, MI 49079
(616) 657-2531

Minnesota
West Central Community Service Center
1125 6th Street, S.E.
Willmar, MN 56201
(612) 235-4613

Ohio
Eastway Corporation
600 Wayne Avenue
Dayton, OH 45410
(513) 222-4900

Woodland Centers, Inc.
412 Vinton Pike
Gallipolis, OH 45631
(614) 446-5500

Oklahoma
Jim Taliaferro Community Mental
  Health Center
602 S.W. 38th Street
Lawton, OK 73505
(405) 248-5780

Oregon
Mount Hood Community Mental
  Health Center
400 N.E. 7th Street
Gresham, OR 97030
(503) 661-5455

Rhode Island
MHS of Cranston, Johnston, and
  Northwest Rhode Island
1516 Atwood Avenue
Johnston, RI 02919
(401) 273-8741

Northern Rhode Island Community
  Mental Health Center
181 Cumberland Street
Woonsocket, RI 02895
(401) 765-8585

Virginia
Alexandria Community Mental Health
  Center
206 North Washington Street, 5th Floor
Alexandria, VA 22314
(703) 836-5751

Comprehensive Mental Health Services
Pembroke Three, Suite 138
Virginia Beach, VA 23462
(804) 490-0583

Washington
Spokane Community Mental Health
Center
South 107 Division
Spokane, WA 99202
(509) 458-7450

Wyoming
Southwest Counseling Service
1124 College Road
Rock Springs, WY 82901
(307) 362-6615

National Association of Social Workers: Chapter Offices

Alabama Chapter, NASW
100 Commerce Street, Suite 407
Montgomery, AL 36104
(205) 263-7060

Alaska Chapter, NASW
8923 Tanis Drive
Juneau, AK 99801
(907) 789-7099

Arizona Chapter, NASW
610 West Broadway, Suite 218
Tempe, AZ 85281
(602) 968-4595

Arkansas Chapter, NASW
1123 South University, Suite 615
Little Rock, AR 72204
(501) 663-0658

California Chapter, NASW
Los Angeles Branch Office
5225 Wilshire Boulevard, Suite 516
Los Angeles, CA 90036
(213) 935-2050

California Chapter, NASW
1225 8th Street, Suite 425
Sacramento, CA 95814
(916) 442-4656

Colorado Chapter, NASW
311 Steele Street, Suite 10
Denver, CO 80206
(303) 399-2782

Connecticut Chapter, NASW
1800 Silas Deane Highway, Suite 20–21
Rocky Hill, CT 06067
(203) 257-8066

Delaware Chapter, NASW
1525 Concord Pike
Wilmington, DE 19803
(302) 654-0999

Metro Washington, District of
Columbia, Chapter, NASW
2025 Eye Street, NW, Suite 105
Washington, DC 20006
(202) 457-0492

Florida Chapter, NASW
345 South Magnolia Drive, No. 14B
Tallahassee, FL 32301
(904) 224-2400

Georgia Chapter, NASW
3166 Maple Drive, N.E., Suite 200-B
Atlanta, GA 30305
(404) 262-1490

Hawaii Chapter, NASW
200 North Vineyard Street, Suite 20
Honolulu, HI 96817
(808) 521-2377; (808) 543-9946

Idaho Chapter, NASW
200 North 4th Street
Boise, ID 83702
(208) 343-2752

Illinois Chapter, NASW
180 North Michigan Avenue, Suite 400
Chicago, IL 60601
(312) 236-8308

Indiana Chapter, NASW
1100 West 42nd Street, Suite 316
Indianapolis, IN 46208
(317) 923-9878

Iowa Chapter, NASW
4211 Grand Avenue
Des Moines, IA 50312
(515) 277-1117

Kansas Chapter, NASW
817 West Sixth Street
Topeka, KS 66603
(913) 354-4804

Kentucky Chapter, NASW
226 B West Second Street,
   P.O. Box 1211
Frankfort, KY 40602
(502) 223-0245

Louisiana Chapter, NASW
LSU School of Social Work
311 Huey Long Field House
Baton Rouge, LA 70803
(504) 388-5437

Maine Chapter, NASW
60 Mabel Street
Portland, ME 04103
(207) 773-1394

Maryland Chapter, NASW
5710 Executive Drive, Suite 105
Baltimore, MD 21228
(301) 788-1066

Massachusetts Chapter, NASW
14 Beacon Street, Suite 409
Boston, MA 02108
(617) 227-9635

Michigan Chapter, NASW
230 North Washington Square,
   Suite 212
Lansing, MI 48933
(517) 487-1548

Minnesota Chapter, NASW
480 Concordia Avenue
St. Paul, MN 55103
(612) 293-1935

Mississippi Chapter, NASW
P.O. Box 4228
Jackson, MS 39216
(601) 981-8359

Missouri Chapter, NASW
Parkade Center, Suite 138
601 Business Loop 70 West
Columbia, MO 65203
(314) 874-6140; (800) 333-6279

Montana Chapter, NASW
20 Hodgeman Canyon
Bozeman, MT 59715
(406) 586-9500

Nebraska Chapter, NASW
6521 Hamilton Street
Omaha, NE 68132
(402) 477-7344

Nevada Chapter, NASW
Box 43, 557 California Street
Boulder City, NV 89005
(702) 293-2087; 293-3911, leave
   message

New Hampshire Chapter, NASW
c/o New Hampshire Association for the
   Blind
25 Walker Street
Concord, NH 03301
(603) 224-4039

New Jersey Chapter, NASW
110 West State Street
Trenton, NJ 08608
(609) 394-1666

New Mexico Chapter, NASW
1503 University Boulevard, N.E.
Albuquerque, NM 87102
(505) 247-2336

New York City Chapter, NASW
545 8th Avenue, 6th Floor
New York, NY 10018
(212) 947-5000

New York State Chapter, NASW
225 Lark Street
Albany, NY 12210
(518) 463-4741; (800) 724-6279

North Carolina Chapter, NASW
P.O. Box 12082
715 West Johnson Street, Suite 204
Raleigh, NC 27605
(919) 828-9650

North Dakota Chapter, NASW
P.O. Box 1775
Jamestown, ND 58502-1775
(701) 223-4161

Ohio Chapter, NASW
40 West Long Street, Suite 203
Columbus, OH 43215
(614) 461-4484

Oklahoma Chapter, NASW
P.O. Box 2609
Norman, OK 73070
(405) 329-7003

Oregon Chapter, NASW
109 N.E. 50th Avenue
Portland, OR 97213
(503) 232-6003

Pennsylvania Chapter, NASW
No. 2 Shore Drive Office Center
2001 North Front Street
Harrisburg, PA 17102
(717) 232-4125

Puerto Rico Chapter, NASW
D-3 Via Bernardo, Monte Alvernia
Rio Piedras, PR 00927
(809) 758-3588

Rhode Island Chapter, NASW
345 Blackstone Boulevard
Providence, RI 02906
(401) 351-4340

South Carolina Chapter, NASW
P.O. Box 5008
Columbia, SC 29250
(803) 256-8406

South Dakota Chapter, NASW
4961 Sheridan Lake Road
Rapid City, SD 57702
(605) 341-0526

Tennessee Chapter, NASW
P.O. Box 25170
Nashville, TN 37202
(615) 352-5777

Texas Chapter, NASW
810 West 11th Street
Austin, TX 78701
(512) 474-1454

Utah Chapter, NASW
University of Utah
Graduate School of Social Work
Salt Lake City, UT 84112
(801) 583-8855

Vermont Chapter, NASW
P.O. Box 147
Woodstock, VT 05091
(802) 457-3645

Virgin Islands Chapter, NASW
P.O. Box 5247, Sunny Isle
Christiansted
St. Croix, U.S. Virgin Islands 00820
(809) 778-7891, 773-7772

Virginia Chapter, NASW
1500 Forest Avenue, Suite 224
Richmond, VA 23288
(804) 282-0788

Washington Chapter, NASW
2366 Eastlake Avenue, East, Suite 236
Seattle, WA 98102
(206) 325-9791

West Virginia Chapter, NASW
1608 Virginia Street, East
Charleston, WV 25311
(304) 343-6141

Wisconsin Chapter, NASW
6414 Copps Avenue, Suite 218
Madison, WI 53716
(608) 222-7566

Wyoming Chapter, NASW
3904 Dillon Avenue
Cheyenne, WY 82001
(307) 632-6366

Europe
European Chapter, NASW
147th Postal Unit, Box R-207
APO, NY 09102
49-6221-37481

National Association of State Units on Aging (NASUA)

NASUA is a membership association of the state units on aging, which are funded under the Older Americans Act. An individual who would like information about services for older persons on the state level, including mental health services for the aging, could contact his or her respective state unit that is listed below.

Alabama
Commission on Aging
Oscar D. Tucker, Executive Director
136 Catoma Street, 2nd Floor
Montgomery, AL 36130
(205) 261-5743

Alaska
Older Alaskans Commission
Constance Sipe, Director
Department of Administration
Pouch C, Mail Station 0209
Juneau, AK 99811-0209
(907) 465-3250

American Samoa
Territorial Administration on Aging
Tali Maae, Director
Office of the Governor
Pago Pago, American Samoa 96799
011 (684) 633-1252

Arizona
Aging and Adult Administration
Richard Littler, Director
Department of Economic Security
1400 West Washington Street
Phoenix, AZ 85007
(602) 255-4446

Arkansas
Division of Aging and Adult Services
Herb Sanderson, Director
Arkansas Department of Human
  Services
1417 Donaghey Plaza South
7th and Main Streets
Little Rock, AR 72201
(501) 682-2441

California
Department of Aging
Alice Gonzales, Director
1600 K Street
Sacramento, CA 95814
(916) 322-5290

Colorado
Aging and Adult Service
Rita Barreras, Manager
Department of Social Services
1575 Sherman Street, 10th Floor
Denver, CO 80203-1714
(303) 866-5931

Connecticut
Department on Aging
Mary Ellen Klinck, Commissioner
175 Main Street
Hartford, CT 06106
(203) 566-3238

Delaware
Division on Aging
Eleanor Cain, Director
Department of Health and Social
  Services
1901 North DuPont Highway
New Castle, DE 19720
(302) 421-6791

District of Columbia
Office on Aging
Veronica Pace, Executive Director
1424 K Street, NW, 2nd Floor
Washington, DC 20005
(202) 724-5626

Florida
Program Office of Aging and Adult Services
Margaret Lynn Duggar, Assistant
  Secretary
Department of Health and
  Rehabilitative Services
1317 Winewood Boulevard
Tallahassee, FL 32301
(904) 488-8922

Georgia
Office of Aging
Fred McGinnis, Director
878 Peachtree Street, N.E., Room 632
Atlanta, GA 30309
(404) 894-5333

Guam
Division of Senior Citizens
Florence P. Shimizu, Administrator
Department of Public Health and Social
  Services
Government of Guam
P.O. Box 2816
Agana, Guam 96910

Hawaii
Executive Office on Aging
Jeanette Takamura, Director
Office of the Governor
335 Merchant Street, Room 241
Honolulu, HI 96813
(808) 548-2593

Idaho
Office on Aging
Charlene Martindale, Director
Room 114, Statehouse
Boise, ID 83720
(208) 334-3833

Illinois
Department on Aging
Janet S. Otwell, Director
421 East Capitol Avenue
Springfield, IL 62701
(217) 785-2870

Indiana
Division on Aging Services
Joyce Smidley, Director
Department of Human Services
251 North Illinois Street, P.O. Box 7083
Indianapolis, IN 46207-7083
(317) 232-7020

Iowa
Department of Elder Affairs
Betty Grandquist, Executive Director
Suite 236, Jewett Building
914 Grand Avenue
Des Moines, IA 50319
(515) 281-5187

Kansas
Department on Aging
Esther Valladolid Wolf, Secretary
Docking State Office Building, 122-S
915 S.W. Harrison
Topeka, KS 66612-1500
(913) 296-4986

Kentucky
Division of Aging Services
Sue Tuttle, Director
Cabinet for Human Resources
CHR Building, 6th West
275 East Main Street
Frankfort, KY 40621
(502) 564-6930

Louisiana
Office of Elderly Affairs
Vickey Hunt, Director
P.O. Box 80374
Baton Rouge, LA 70898
(504) 925-1700

Maine
Bureau of Maine's Elderly
Christine Gianopoulos, Director
Department of Human Services
State House, Station No. 11
Augusta, ME 04333
(207) 289-2561

Mariana Islands
Office of Elderly Programs
Augustine Moses, Acting Chief
Community Development Division
Government of TTPI
Saipan, Mariana Islands 96950
Tel. nos. 9335 or 9336

Maryland
Office on Aging
Rosalie Abrams, Director
State Office Building
301 West Preston Street, Room 1004
Baltimore, MD 21201
(301) 225-1100

Massachusetts
Executive Office of Elder Affairs
Paul J. Lanzikos, Secretary
38 Chauncey Street
Boston, MA 02111
(617) 727-7750

Michigan
Office of Services to the Aging
Olivia Maynard, Director
P.O. Box 30026
Lansing, MI 48909
(517) 373-8230

Minnesota
Board on Aging
Gerald Bloedow, Executive Director
Human Services Building
444 Lafayette Road, 4th Floor
St. Paul, MN 55155-3843
(612) 296-2770

Mississippi
Council on Aging
David K. Brown, Director
301 West Pearl Street
Jackson, MS 39203-3092
(601) 949-2070

Missouri
Division on Aging
Edwin Walker, Director
Department of Social Services
2701 West Main Street, P.O. Box 1337
Jefferson City, MO 65102
(314) 751-3082

Montana
Department of Family Services
Eugene Huntington, Director
48 North Last Chance Gulch,
   P.O. Box 8005
Helena, MT 59604
(406) 444-5900

Nebraska
Department on Aging
Betsy Palmer, Director
301 Centennial Mall, South
P.O. Box 95044
Lincoln, NE 68509
(402) 471-2306

Nevada
Division for Aging Services
Suzanne Ernst, Administrator
Department of Human Resources
340 North 11th Street
Las Vegas, NV 89101
(702) 486-3545

New Hampshire
Division of Elderly and Adult Services
Richard Chevrefils, Director
6 Hazen Drive
Concord, NH 03301-6501
(603) 271-4680

New Jersey
Division on Aging
Ann Zahora, Director
Department of Community Affairs
CN807 South Broad and Front Streets
Trenton, NJ 08625-0807
(609) 292-4833

New Mexico
State Agency on Aging
Stephanie Fallcreek, Director
224 East Palace Avenue, 4th Floor
La Villa Rivera Building
Santa Fe, NM 87501
(505) 827-7640

New York
Office for the Aging
Jane Gould, Acting Director
New York State Plaza
Agency Building No. 2
Albany, NY 12223
(518) 474-4425

North Carolina
Division of Aging
Alfred B. Boyles, Director
1985 Umstead Drive, Kirby Building
Raleigh, NC 27603
(919) 733-3983

North Dakota
Aging Services
Larry Brewster, Administrator
Department of Human Services
State Capitol Building
Bismarck, ND 58505
(701) 224-2577

Northern Mariana Islands
Office on Aging
Edward Cabrera, Administrator
Department of Community and Cultural
   Affairs
Civic Center–Susupe
Saipan, Northern Mariana Islands 96950
Tel. nos. 9411 or 9732

Ohio
Department of Aging
Carol Austin, Director
50 West Broad Street, 9th Floor
Columbus, OH 43266-0501
(614) 466-5500

Oklahoma
Aging Services Division
Roy Keen, Division Administrator
Department of Human Services
P.O. Box 25352
Oklahoma City, OK 73125
(405) 521-2281

Oregon
Senior Services Division
Richard Ladd, Administrator
313 Public Service Building
Salem, OR 97310
(503) 378-4728

Pennsylvania
Department of Aging
Linda Rhodes, Secretary
231 State Street
Harrisburg, PA 17101-1195
(717) 783-1550

Puerto Rico
Gericulture Commission
Celia E. Cintron, Executive Director
Department of Social Services
Apartado 11398
Santurce, PR 00910
(809) 721-4010

Rhode Island
Department of Elderly Affairs
Adelaide Luber, Director
79 Washington Street
Providence, RI 02903
(401) 277-2858

South Carolina
Commission on Aging
Ruth Seigler, Director
400 Arbor Lake Drive, Suite B-500
Columbia, SC 29223
(803) 735-0210

South Dakota
Office of Adult Services and Aging
Michael Vogel, Executive Director
700 North Illinois Street
Kneip Building
Pierre, SD 57501
(605) 773-3656

Tennessee
Commission on Aging
Emily Wiseman, Executive Director
706 Church Street, Suite 201
Nashville, TN 37219-5573
(615) 741-2056

Texas
Department on Aging
O. P. (Bob) Bobbitt, Director
P.O. Box 12786, Capitol Station
1949 IH-35, South
Austin, TX 78741-3702
(512) 444-2727

Utah
Division of Aging and Adult Services
Robert K. Ward, Director
Department of Social Services
120 North, 200 West
Box 45500
Salt Lake City, UT 84145-0500
(801) 538-3910

Vermont
Office on Aging
Joel Cook, Director
103 South Main Street
Waterbury, VT 05676
(802) 241-2400

Virgin Islands
Department of Human Services
Grace Joseph, Assistant Administrator
6F Havensight Mall–Charlotte Amalie
St. Thomas, Virgin Islands 00801
(809) 774-5884

Virginia
Department for the Aging
Wilda Ferguson, Commissioner
700 Centre, 10th Floor
700 East Franklin Street
Richmond, VA 23219-2327
(804) 225-2271

Washington
Aging and Adult Services
   Administration
Charles Reed, Assistant Secretary
Department of Social and Health
   Services, OB-44A
Olympia, WA 98504
(206) 586-3768

West Virginia
Commission on Aging
Susan Harman, Director
Holly Grove, State Capitol
Charleston, WV 25305
(304) 348-3317

Wisconsin
Bureau of Aging
Donna McDowell, Director
Division of Community Services
One West Wilson Street, Room 480
Madison, WI 53702
(608) 266-2536

Wyoming
Commission on Aging
Scott Sessions, Director
Hathaway Building, Room 139
Cheyenne, WY 82002-0710
(307) 777-7986

National Mental Health Association:
Affiliated Divisions/Chapters

Alabama
Mental Health Association in Alabama
306 Whitman Street
Montgomery, AL 36104
(205) 834-3857

Alaska
Alaska Mental Health Association
4050 Lake Otis Parkway, Suite 202
Anchorage, AK 99508
(907) 563-0880

Arizona
Mental Health Association in Arizona
P.O. Box 37071
Tucson, AZ 85740

Arkansas
Mental Health Association in Northwest
   Arkansas
P.O. Box 1993
Fayetteville, AR 72702
(501) 521-1158

California
Mental Health Association in California
926 J Street, Suite 611
Sacramento, CA 95814
(916) 441-4627

Florida
Mental Health Association of Florida
2337 Wednesday Street
Tallahassee, FL 32308
(904) 385-7527

Georgia
Mental Health Association of Georgia
1244 Clairmont Road, Suite 204
Decatur, GA 30030
(404) 634-2850

Hawaii
Mental Health Association of Hawaii
200 North Vineyard Boulevard, No. 507
Honolulu, HI 96817
(808) 521-1846

Idaho
Mental Health Association in Idaho
715 South Capitol Boulevard, Suite 401
Boise, ID 83702
(208) 343-4866

Kentucky
Kentucky Mental Health Association
400 Sherburn Lane, Suite 357
Louisville, KY 40207
(502) 893-0460

Louisiana
Mental Health Association of Louisiana
6700 Plaza Drive, Suite 104
New Orleans, LA 70127
(504) 241-3462

Maryland
Mental Health Association of Maryland
323 East 25th Street, 2nd Floor
Baltimore, MD 21218
(301) 235-1178

Michigan
Mental Health Association in Michigan
15920 West Twelve Mile Road
Southfield, MI 48076
(313) 557-6777

Nebraska
Mental Health Association in Nebraska
4600 Valley Road, Room 411
Lincoln, NE 68510
(402) 488-1080

New Jersey
Mental Health Association in New
  Jersey
60 South Fullerton Avenue, Room 105
Montclair, NJ 07042
(201) 744-2500

New York
Mental Health Association in New York
  State
75 New Scotland Avenue
Albany, NY 12208
(518) 434-0439

North Carolina
Mental Health Association in North
  Carolina
115 1/2 West Morgan Street
Raleigh, NC 27601
(919) 828-8145

Oklahoma
Mental Health Association in Oklahoma
  County
5104 North Francis, Suite B (Shartel
  Shopping Center)
Oklahoma City, OK 73118
(405) 524-6363

Mental Health Association in Tulsa
1502 South Denver
Tulsa, OK 74119
(918) 585-1213

Rhode Island
Mental Health Association of Rhode
  Island
855 Waterman Avenue, Suite D
East Providence, RI 02914
(401) 431-1240

South Carolina
Mental Health Association in South
  Carolina
1823 Gadsden Street
Columbia, SC 29201
(803) 779-5363

Tennessee
Mental Health Association in Tennessee
1844 Stonebrook Drive
Knoxville, TN 37923
(615) 637-8210, 690-1175

Texas
Mental Health Association in Texas
8401 Shoal Creek Boulevard
Austin, TX 78758
(512) 454-3706

Utah
Mental Health Association in Utah
255 East 400 South, Suite 150
Salt Lake City, UT 84111
(801) 531-8996

Self-Help Clearinghouses

Self-help clearinghouses offer assistance in locating local and national self-help groups and organizations devoted to addressing the needs of people with a wide variety of concerns.

Arizona
Rainy Day People Project (in
    development)
Pat Becker, Founder
P.O. Box 472
Scottsdale, AZ 85252

California
Bay Area Self-Help Center
Mental Health Association
2398 Pine Street
San Francisco, CA 94115
(415) 921-4401

California Self-Help Center
Fran Dory, Director
U.C.L.A. Psychology Department
405 Hilgard Avenue
Los Angeles, CA 90024
(213) 825-1799; in California (800)
    222-LINK

Central Valley Self-Help Center
Geri Stewart, Coordinator
Mental Health Association
P.O. Box 343
Merced, CA 95341
(209) 723-8861

Northern Region Self-Help Center
Pat Camper, Coordinator
Mental Health Association
5370 Elvas Avenue, Suite B
Sacramento, CA 95819
(916) 456-2070

Self-Help Clearinghouse of Yolo County
Elaine Talley, Director
Mental Health Association
P.O. Box 447
Davis, CA 95617
(916) 756-8181

Southern Region Self-Help Center
Mental Health Association of San Diego
3958 Third Avenue
San Diego, CA 92103

Connecticut
Connecticut Self-Help/Mutual Support
    Network
Vicki Spiro Smith, Coordinator
Consultation Center
19 Howe Street
New Haven, CT 06511
(203) 789-7645

District of Columbia
Self-Help Clearinghouse of Greater
  Washington (Washington, D.C.,
  northern Virginia, and southern
  Maryland)
Kim Haines
Mental Health Association of Northern
  Virginia
100 North Washington Street, Suite 232
Falls Church, VA 22046
(703) 536-4100

Illinois
Self-Help Center
Family Service of Champaign County
405 South State Street
Champaign, IL 61820
(217) 352-0092

Self-Help Center
Daryl Isenberg, Director
1600 Dodge Avenue, Suite S-122
Evanston, IL 60201
(312) 328-0470; in Illinois (800)
  322-M.A.S.H.

Iowa
Iowa Self-Help Clearinghouse
Carla Lawson, Director
Iowa Pilot Parents, Inc.
33 North 12th Street
Fort Dodge, IA 50501
(515) 576-5870; in Iowa (800)
  383-4777

Kansas
Self-Help Network
David F. Gleason, Director
Campus Box 34
Wichita State University
Wichita, KS 67208-1595
(316) 689-3170

Massachusetts
Massachusetts Clearinghouse of Mutual
  Help Groups
Warren Schumacher, Director
Massachusetts Cooperative Extension
113 Skinner Hall
University of Massachusetts
Amherst, MA 01003
(413) 545-2313

Michigan
Center for Self-Help
Pat Friend and Rob Hess
Riverwood Center
1485 Highway M-139
Benton Harbor, MI 49022
(616) 925-0594

Michigan Self-Help Clearinghouse
Toni Young, Coordinator
Michigan Protection and Advocacy
  Service
109 West Michigan Avenue, Suite 900
Lansing, MI 48933
(517) 484-7373; in Michigan (800)
  752-5858

Minnesota
Minnesota Mutual Help Resource
  Center
Wilder Foundation Community Care
  Unit
919 Lafond Avenue
St. Paul, MN 55104
(612) 642-4060

Missouri
Support Group Clearinghouse
Becky Brozovich, Coordinator
Kansas City Association for Mental
  Health
1020 East 63rd Street
Kansas City, MO 64110
(816) 561-HELP

Nebraska
Self-Help Information Services
Barbara Fox, Director; Joyce Burgess,
    Information Specialist
1601 Euclid Avenue
Lincoln, NE 68502
(402) 476-9668

New Jersey
New Jersey Self-Help Clearinghouse
Edward J. Madara, Director; Toni Ross,
    Program Coordinator; Abbie Meese,
    Information Referral Service
    Coordinator
Saint Clares–Riverside Medical Center
Denville, NJ 07834
(201) 625-9565; TDD (201) 625-9053;
    in New Jersey (800) FOR-MASH
    (mutual aid self-help)

New York
Brooklyn Self-Help Clearinghouse
Carol Berkvist, Director
Heights Hills Mental Health Service
30 Third Avenue
Brooklyn, NY 11217
(718) 834-7341, 834-7332

Long Island Self-Help Clearinghouse
Pat Verdino, Director
New York Institute of Technology
Central Islip Campus
Central Islip, NY 11722
(516) 348-3030

New York City Self-Help Clearinghouse,
    Inc.
P.O. Box 022812
Brooklyn, NY 11202
(718) 596-6000

New York State Self-Help Clearinghouse
Mary Huber, Director
New York Council of Children & Families
Empire State Plaza, Tower 2
Albany, NY 12224
(518) 474-6293

Westchester Self-Help Clearinghouse
Leslie Borck, Director; Lenore
    Rosenbaum, Coordinator
Westchester Community College
Academic Arts Building
75 Grasslands Road
Valhalla, NY 10595
(914) 347-3620

Oregon
Northwest Regional Self-Help
    Clearinghouse
Doreen Akkerman, Coordinator
718 West Burnside Street
Portland, OR 97209
(503) 222-5555 information & referrals,
    226-9360 administrative

Pennsylvania
Self-Help Group Network of the
    Pittsburgh Area
Betty Hepner, Coordinator
710¹/₂ South Avenue
Wilkensburg, PA 15221
(412) 247-5400

S.H.I.N.E. (Self-Help Information
    Network Exchange)
Eric Fetterolf, Director
c/o Voluntary Action Center
225 North Washington Avenue
Park Plaza, Lower Level
Scranton, PA 18503
(717) 961-1234

Rhode Island
Support Group Helpline
Deborah Reavey, Contact Person
Rhode Island Department of Health
Cannon Building
Davis Street
Providence, RI 02908
(401) 277-2231

South Carolina
Midland Area Support Group Network
Mary Burton, Coordinator
Lexington Medical Center
2720 Sunset Boulevard
West Columbia, SC 29169
(803) 791-9227

Tennessee
Support Group Clearinghouse
Judy Balloff, Program Coordinator
Mental Health Association of Knox
  County
6712 Kingston Pike, No. 203
Knoxville, TN 37919
(614) 584-6736

Texas
Dallas Self-Help Clearinghouse
Carol Madison, Director
Mental Health Association of Dallas
  County
2500 Maple Avenue
Dallas, TX 75201-1998
(214) 871-2420

Greater San Antonio Self-Help
  Clearinghouse
Mental Health in Greater San Antonio
1407 North Main
San Antonio, TX 78212
(512) 222-1571

Self-Help Clearinghouse
Dianne Long, Coordinator
Mental Health Association in Houston
  & Harris County
2211 Norfolk, Suite 810
Houston, TX 77098
(713) 523-8963

Tarrant County Self-Help Clearinghouse
Mental Health Association of Tarrant
  County
3136 West 4th Street
Fort Worth, TX 76107-2113
(817) 335-5405

Texas Self-Help Clearinghouse
Mental Health Association in Texas
1111 West 24th Street
Austin, TX 78705
(512) 454-3706

Vermont
Vermont Self-Help Clearinghouse
Donna Carpenter, Coordinator
c/o Parents Assistance Line
103 South Main Street
Waterbury, VT 05676
(802) 241-2249; in Vermont (800)
  442-5356

U.S. National Self-Help Organizations

National Self-Help Clearinghouse
Frank Riessman, Director
City University of New York Graduate
  Center, Room 1206A
33 West 42nd Street
New York, NY 10036
(212) 840-1259

Self-Help Center
Daryl Isenberg, Director
1600 Dodge Avenue, Suite S-122
Evanston, IL 60201
(312) 328-0470

Self-Help Clearinghouse
Edward J. Madara, Department Director
Saint Clares–Riverside Medical Center
Denville, NJ 07834
(201) 625-9565; TDD (201) 625-9053

Canada

Family Life Education Council
Sonia Eisler, Executive Director
233 12th Avenue S.W.
Calgary, Alberta, Canada T2R 0G9
(403) 262-1117

Self-Help Collaboration Project
Barbara Grantham, Manager
United Way of the Lower Mainland
1625 West 8th Avenue
Vancouver, British Columbia, Canada
 V6J 1T9
(604) 731-7781

Winnipeg Self-Help Resource
 Clearinghouse
Bernice Marmel, Director
NorWest Coop & Health Center
103-61 Tyndall Avenue
Winnipeg, Manitoba, Canada R2X 2T4
(204) 589-5500, 633-5955

Canadian Council on Social Development
Conseil Canadien de Developpement
 Social
Hector Balthazar
P.O. Box 3505, Station C
Ottawa, Ontario, Canada K1Y 4G1
(613) 728-1865

Self-Help Clearinghouse of
 Metropolitan Toronto
Lori Kociol, Director
40 Orchard View Boulevard, Suite 215
Toronto, Ontario, Canada M4R 1B9
(416) 487-4355

CAMAC—Centre d'Aide Mutuelle, Inc.
M. Jean-Claude Boisvert, President
C.P. 535, Succ. Desjardins
Montreal, Quebec, Canada H5B 1B6
(514) 341-1440

Self-Help Development Unit
Sharon Miller, Coordinator
410 Cumberland Avenue North
Saskatoon, Saskatchewan, Canada
 S7M 1M6
(306) 652-7817

Chapter 6

Reference Materials

Books

The following is a selective annotated bibliography of books on aging and/or mental health. The first section lists books that may be of interest to professionals who want to acquaint themselves with topics in mental health and aging. The second section reviews books that are appropriate for the general public and is divided into books dealing with general issues on aging, general issues on mental health, and the specific topic of mental health and aging.

Books for the Professional

Binstock, Robert H., and Linda K. George, eds. *Handbook of Aging and the Social Sciences*. 3d ed. New York: Academic Press, 1989. 454p. $65. ISBN 0-12-099190-X.

> This is one of a set of three handbooks on aging, all of which are now in the third edition. The handbooks are critical and authoritative reviews of scientific and professional literature on different topics in aging. They are written by persons who are prominent in their respective fields. The handbooks are a major resource for those seeking a scholarly overview of different issues in gerontology. The *Handbook of Aging and the Social Sciences* examines general issues in aging and social structure, aging and the life course, aging and social institutions, and aging and social interventions. Although there are no chapters that directly discuss mental health, the book offers an important review of the social context of late-life emotional adjustment.

Birren, James E., and K. Warner Schaie, eds. *Handbook of the Psychology of Aging.* 3d ed. New York: Academic Press, 1989. 501p. $65. ISBN 0-12-101280-8.

> This is also one of the set of three handbooks on aging (see previous listing). The *Handbook of the Psychology of Aging* reviews a breadth of topics including theory and measurement in the psychology of aging, influences of behavior and aging, behavioral processes in aging, and application of psychology to the individual and society. Although only four chapters address mental health issues, the book is an important resource. Previous editions of this and other handbooks may also be of interest.

Birren, James E., and R. Bruce Sloane, eds. *Handbook of Mental Health and Aging.* Englewood Cliffs, NJ: Prentice-Hall, 1980. 1064p. $105. ISBN 0-13-380261-2.

> This is a very large collection of chapters on various aspects of mental health and aging including the neurosciences, behavioral sciences, and social sciences; diagnostic issues; treatment; and prevention. At this point some of the chapters are dated and better summaries are available elsewhere. Other chapters within the book are still fairly current.

Breslau, Lawrence D., and Marie R. Haug, eds. *Depression and Aging: Causes, Care, and Consequences.* New York: Springer, 1983. 352p. $26.95. ISBN 0-8261-3710-5.

> This is a collection of essays on the etiology, diagnosis, treatment, and consequences of depression in older adults. The quality of the chapters varies. The book contains a fairly good bibliography although it is now a bit dated.

Busse, Ewald W., and Dan G. Blazer, eds. *Geriatric Psychiatry.* Washington, DC: American Psychiatric Press, 1989. 725p. $55. ISBN 0-88048-279-6.

> *Geriatric Psychiatry* contains 25 chapters on the theory and practice of geriatric psychiatry. The book examines social, psychological, and biological issues that bear on late-life mental health; diagnostic issues; and the nature and treatment of major psychiatric disorders. The chapters are written by persons prominent in their areas of expertise. This is probably one of the best existing books on geriatric psychiatry.

Butler, Robert N., and Myrna I. Lewis. *Aging and Mental Health: Positive Psychosocial and Biomedical Approaches.* 3d ed. Columbus, OH: Merrill, 1982. 483p. $26.95 (paperback). ISBN 0-675-20920-X.

> The senior author of this book is a psychiatrist and first director of the National Institute on Aging. The book discusses the circumstances of later life, the problems of older adults, and the evaluation, treatment, and prevention of late-life mental health problems. Like Dr. Butler's book *Why Survive: Being Old in America,* the volume is critical of larger social forces and government policies that negatively influence the mental health of the aged in the United States. A fourth edition of this book is expected in 1990.

Carstensen, Laura L., and Barry A. Edelstein, eds. *Handbook of Clinical Gerontology.* New York: Pergamon Press, 1987. 448p. $75. ISBN 0-08-031947-5.

> This collection reviews select issues in normal aging, the nature of major mental disorders in older adults, common medical problems of late life, and some social factors that bear on late-life adjustment. It is a generally good book although some chapters are less well researched and written than others.

Chaisson-Stewart, Maureen G., ed. *Depression in the Elderly: An Interdisciplinary Approach.* New York: Wiley, 1985. 377p. $25. ISBN 0-471-87059-5.

> This is a detailed look at a wide variety of issues related to depression in later life. The book includes biological, social, and psychological perspectives on depression. Although chiefly oriented for professionals, it is written clearly enough that a motivated nonprofessional would be able to follow the topics it discusses.

Edinberg, Mark. *Mental Health Practice with the Elderly.* Englewood Cliffs, NJ: Prentice-Hall, 1985. 320p. $43.20. ISBN 0-13-575994-3.

> This is a review and integration of a variety of issues that bear on mental health in older adults. The book is directed to mental health professionals of various disciplines and would be useful both for those familiar and for those unfamiliar with the topic. The book is composed of four sections that respectively address the processes of aging, psychopathology and assessment, intervention

with older adults, and the delivery of mental health services. This is a thorough and well-written book by a psychologist familiar with both the academic and applied aspects of the field of aging.

Gwyther, Lisa P. *Care of Alzheimer's Patients: A Manual for Nursing Home Staff.* Co-published by the American Health Care Association and the Alzheimer's Disease and Related Disorders Association, 1985. 122p. $6.95 (paperback). Available from: The Alzheimer's Association, 70 East Lake Street, Chicago, IL 60601; (800) 621-0379, in Illinois (800) 572-6037.

> This book was authored by a social worker with considerable knowledge and experience in the care of persons with dementia. The volume is very clearly written and offers valuable suggestions on how to deal with the myriad problems that nursing home staff confront in caring for persons with dementia. Topics covered include problems of wandering, suspiciousness, inappropriate behavior, and depression. The book frequently uses clinical vignettes. Although directed to nursing home personnel, it is useful for other professionals and for family members of dementia patients.

Jarvik, Lissy F., and Carol H. Winograd, eds. *Treatment for the Alzheimer Patient: The Long Haul.* New York: Springer, 1988. 288p. $29.95. ISBN 0-8261-6000-X.

> In an effort to combat the "therapeutic nihilism" that is commonly expressed about dementia patients by some health care personnel, the editors have gathered a series of papers that address what *can* be done. Chapters of this book recommend efforts that can be made by physicians, psychiatrists, nurses, psychologists, social workers, and other health professionals to help dementia patients and their families to better cope with cognitive decline.

Jenike, Michael A. *Handbook of Geriatric Psychopharmacology.* Littleton, MA: PSG Publishing Company, 1985. 178p. $20. ISBN 0-88416-520-5.

> This is a review of issues involved in prescribing psychotropic medications to older adults. It discusses differences in drug metabolism between younger and older adults and suggests strategies for prescribing specific psychotropic medications for older individuals.

Johnson, Colleen L., and Leslie A. Grant. *The Nursing Home in American Society*. Baltimore, MD: The Johns Hopkins University Press, 1985. 208p. $24.50. ISBN 0-8018-2502-4. $10.95 (paperback). ISBN 0-8018-2503-2.

> This volume describes the U.S. nursing home: routes to entry, life within, and policy issues that affect it. This scholarly introduction to the topic will be useful for researchers, practitioners, and nonprofessionals who desire a general understanding of the function of long-term care facilities in this country. It includes a discussion of the mental health needs of nursing home residents. The book contains a fairly extensive bibliography.

Kermis, Marguerite D. *Mental Health in Late Life: The Adaptive Process*. Boston and Monterey, CA: Jones and Bartlett, 1986. 392p. $22.50. ISBN 0-86720-353-6.

> This is a readable and well-researched book that deals with a wide variety of issues that bear on mental health in late life. There is a strong spirit of advocacy in the book (similar to that in works by Robert Butler). The author is particularly critical of existing systems of mental health care for the aged. This is a good resource for the mental health professional who wants detailed and thoughtful coverage of issues on mental health and the elderly.

Knight, Bob. *Psychotherapy with Older Adults*. Beverly Hills, CA: Sage Publications, 1986. 240p. $25. ISBN 0-8039-2633-2.

> This book is written by a psychologist with extensive experience in the delivery of mental health services to the aged. It examines critical issues in doing psychotherapy with older people and provides clear and practical advice on how to engage and treat the older client. It is one of the best existing books on psychotherapy with the aged.

Lazarus, Lawrence W., ed. *Essentials of Geriatric Psychiatry: A Guide for Health Professionals*. New York: Springer, 1988. 272p. $29.95. ISBN 0-8261-5990-7.

> This book is sponsored by the American Association for Geriatric Psychiatry, a professional organization of psychiatrists who provide care to older adults. Chapters are written by different persons with expertise in geriatric psychiatry and cover a range

of topics. The main focus of the book, however, is on the diagnosis and treatment of mental disorders in the aged. Book chapters are written in outline form.

Lurie, Elinor E., and James H. Swan, eds. *Serving the Mentally Ill Elderly: Problems and Perspectives*. Lexington, MA: Lexington Books, 1987. 352p. $35. ISBN 0-669-14113-5.

> This volume examines a variety of topics in mental health and aging including epidemiology, the interrelationship between physical and mental illness, the effectiveness of treatments for mental disorders in the aged, the mental health system, reimbursement of mental health services, and self-help organizations for the aged. The book will be especially helpful for research-oriented professionals seeking a good critical evaluation of research on mental health and aging.

Miller, Nancy E., and Gene D. Cohen, eds. *Schizophrenia and Aging: Schizophrenia, Paranoia, and Schizophreniform Disorders in Later Life*. New York: Guilford Press, 1987. 367p. $40. ISBN 0-89862-228-X.

> For individuals with research interests in late-life psychotic illness, this is *the* book to obtain. Chapters address questions about late-life psychoses, about which little is known. Many of the chapters are written by well-known scholars and practitioners.

National Council of Community Mental Health Centers. *Serving the Elderly: A Mental Health Resource Guide*. National Council of Community Mental Health Centers, 1989. (Published as a part of the series On the Cutting Edge: A Series of Community Mental Health Program Models.) 127p. $45 (paperback) for nonmembers. Available from: The National Council of Community Mental Health Centers, 12300 Twinbrook Parkway, Suite 320, Rockville, MD 20852.

> This is a unique and useful resource book. In Part One, information gleaned from in-depth interviews with personnel from 23 model agencies that provide services to the aged is summarized. Characteristics of the agencies, their service delivery practices, and barriers to service delivery to older adults are discussed. The names, addresses, and phone numbers of the 23 model agencies are included. (Note: The names and addresses of these agencies are provided in Chapter 5 in the section titled "State and Local Resources.") In Part Two, there is a general review of literature

on prevalence of mental disorders in older adults, patterns of service use by older adults, treatment modalities, family issues, and system issues that bear on delivery of services to this population. Part Three contains an annotated bibliography of literature on mental health and aging drawn from the American Psychological Association's databases. This is highly recommended for professionals who provide mental health services to older people.

O'Conner, Kathleen, and Joyce Prothero, eds. *The Alzheimer Caregiver: Strategies for Support.* Seattle: University of Washington Press, 1986. 150p. $20. ISBN 0-295-96385-9. $8.95 (paperback). ISBN 0-295-96346-8.

> This volume describes the nature and diagnosis of Alzheimer's disease and the issues faced by family members caring for individuals with the disease. Although appropriate for professionals who want an introduction to Alzheimer's disease, the book may also be useful for nonprofessionals. It is generally written in nontechnical language.

Salzman, Carl. *Clinical Geriatric Psychopharmacology,* New York: McGraw-Hill, 1984. 248p. $35. ISBN 0-07-054502-2.

> *Clinical Geriatric Psychopharmacology* discusses a variety of issues that bear on prescribing psychotropic medications to older adults. It reviews the relationship between aging and response to psychotropic medications and suggests how the psychiatrist can safely and effectively prescribe psychotropic medications. The book also includes a chapter with information about prescribing and drug interactions. This is a good volume for psychiatrists who prescribe psychotropic medications to older individuals.

Smyer, Michael A., and Margaret Gatz, eds. *Mental Health and Aging: Programs and Evaluations.* Beverly Hills, CA: Sage Publications, 1983. 320p. $29.95. ISBN 0-8039-2100-4. $14.95 (paperback). ISBN 0-8039-2101-2.

> This volume contains a series of papers on mental health–related interventions for older individuals. It includes descriptions of both traditional (e.g., a day treatment program) and nontraditional (e.g., a companion animal program) ways to help older persons. Training programs for those who work with the aged are also described. A useful aspect of this book is that the effectiveness of each of the interventions was systematically evaluated.

Smyer, Michael A., Margaret D. Cohn, and Diane Brannon, eds. *Mental Health Consultation in Nursing Homes*. New York: New York University Press, 1989. 304p. $28. ISBN 0-8147-7879-8.

> Conceptualizing the nursing home as a community of residents, family members, and staff, this book addresses the complex problems and potential of the nursing home. The authors offer their views on the role of the mental health professional in meeting both the needs of the individual nursing home residents and the needs of the larger nursing home community. This is a thoughtful book on a much-neglected topic.

Zarit, Steven H. *Aging and Mental Disorders: Psychological Approaches to Assessment and Treatment*. New York: Free Press, 1980. 454p. $24.95. ISBN 0-02-935850-7.

> This book represented the first serious effort to review and integrate psychological theory and practice as they relate to the mental health problems of the aged. It reviews general issues in aging that bear on mental health, psychopathology in late life, and different treatment approaches. Although the book is a bit dated, it is nevertheless an excellent resource for the clinical gerontologist.

Zarit, Steven H., Nancy K. Orr, and Judy M. Zarit. *The Hidden Victims of Alzheimer's Disease: Families under Stress*. New York: New York University Press, 1985. 224p. $32. ISBN 0-8147-9662-1. $14.95 (paperback). ISBN 0-8147-9663-X.

> This book outlines the authors' program for providing psychological and social support to family members caring for persons with dementia. It also discusses basic issues in the causes and diagnosis of dementia. It is a clear and well-written volume that will be useful to mental health professionals who work with families of dementia patients.

Books for the General Public

GENERAL READING ON AGING

Butler, Robert N. *Why Survive? Being Old in America*. New York: Harper & Row, 1985. 510p. $9.95 (paperback). ISBN 0-06-131997-X.

This is a classic treatise on aging in U.S. society written by the first director of the National Institute on Aging. It explores the social, psychological, economic, psychiatric, medical, and public policy factors that bear on aging. It is a forceful and compassionate book that condemns the mistreatment of older adults and offers a different vision of life for the elderly of the United States. Although the hardcover version of the book was published in the mid-1970s, it should be on the bookshelf of anyone with an interest in gerontology.

Cole, Thomas R., and Sally A. Gadow, eds. *What Does It Mean To Grow Old? Reflections from the Humanities.* Durham, NC: Duke University Press, 1986. 302p. $39.50. ISBN 0-8223-0545-3.

The book is a series of essays originally presented at a conference on aging and meaning. The essays, written by people from many disciplines, draw upon religious, cultural, individual, philosophical, and literary perspectives to grapple with the meaning of late life. The book also includes valuable bibliographic information on this topic. Although directed toward a professional audience, the book should be appealing to nonprofessionals interested in exploring the topic of aging from a humanistic perspective.

Edinberg, Mark. *Talking with Your Aging Parents.* Boston: Shambhala Publications, 1988. 220p. $9.95. ISBN 0-87773-390-2 (paperback).

This book was written by a practicing psychologist who is familiar with the problems of older adults and their families. The book is directed to adult children who want to improve the way they communicate with their elderly parents. The book provides basic and important information on effective communication skills and offers specific suggestions on how to deal with a variety of issues that sometimes create difficulties between parent and adult child. Issues addressed include housing, social matters, legal and financial issues, health and well-being, confusion, death and dying, nursing homes and long-term care, family matters, and the life of the adult child him- or herself. Many useful examples of problems and effective problem-solving efforts are provided. This book is highly recommended.

Erikson, Erik H., with Joan M. Erikson and Helen Q. Kivnick. *Vital Involvement in Old Age.* New York: W. W. Norton, 1986. $19.95. 352p. ISBN 0-393-02359-1. $10.95 (paper). ISBN 0-393-30509-0.

This book was written by one of the foremost U.S. psychoanalysts—Erik Erikson—his wife Joan, and a colleague. Erikson uses his theory of life stages to explore late-life issues faced by a group of octogenarians who, as younger adults, had taken part in a psychological study from which the authors draw material. It is a psychological and poetic book that may appeal to those interested in issues of meaning in later life.

Jarvik, Lissy, and Gary Small. *Parentcare: A Commonsense Guide for Adult Children*. New York: Crown Publishers, 1988. 309p. $19.95. ISBN 0-517-56765-2.

The senior author of *Parentcare* is a prominent researcher in the field of aging. The book addresses emotional and psychological issues commonly confronted by adult children caring for aging parents. It also provides information on a variety of topics (e.g., health, nutrition, sexuality, retirement, and housing) that will be of considerable use to persons unfamiliar with the landscape of late life. Included in the work are a large appendix that outlines common health problems, a description of what different health care professionals do, information on psychotropic drugs, a sample will, the location of regional geriatric programs, and a list of national organizations for the aged.

Schaie, K. Warner, and Sherry L. Willis. *Adult Development and Aging*. 2d ed. Boston: Little, Brown and Company, 1986. 553p. Contact publisher for cost. ISBN 0-673-39090-X.

This is an undergraduate textbook on aging. Both authors are highly respected psychologists who have done pioneering research on the psychology of aging. For nonprofessionals interested in a more scholarly, yet highly readable, approach to issues in adult development and aging, this is a good resource.

Skinner, B. F., and M. E. Vaughan. *Enjoy Old Age: A Program of Self-Management*. New York: W. W. Norton, 1983. 157p. $11.95. ISBN 0-393-01805-9. Also published by New York: Warner Books, 1985. 157p. $5.95 (paperback). ISBN 0-446-38087-3.

Enjoy Old Age is a series of essays by noted psychologist B. F. Skinner and a colleague on how to better manage common challenges of late life. Challenges addressed include limitations of vision, hearing, and memory; excess time; obstacles in the physical environment; changing social roles vis-à-vis friends and family; and emotional distress. The book, printed in large type, is written in easy-to-understand language. The tone is optimistic and the writing is punctuated with gentle humor about the vicissitudes of being an old person.

GENERAL MENTAL HEALTH

Bernheim, Kayla F., Richard R. J. Lewine, and Caroline T. Beale. *The Caring Family: Living with Chronic Mental Illness.* Chicago: Contemporary Books, 1983. 226p. $8.95 (paperback). ISBN 0-8092-5534-0.

> This is a book for family members of persons with mental illness that offers facts, practical advice, and support. It also offers specific suggestions on how to manage problematic behaviors evidenced by the patient, ways to negotiate the mental health system, how to better to deal with legal and financial issues, and techniques for reducing the stresses of patient care.

Committee on Psychiatry and the Community Group for the Advancement of Psychiatry. *A Family Affair: Helping Families Cope with Mental Illness.* New York: Bruner/Mazel, 1986. 110p. $17.95. ISBN 0-87630-444-7. $12.50 (paper). ISBN 0-87630-443-9.

> This book sensitively tells the stories of family members of persons with mental illness. The stories come from letters to Abigail Van Buren, who invited readers of her "Dear Abby" column to share their experiences. It also offers suggestions and insights for those caring for mentally ill persons on how to better manage their complex lives. The book contains a good list of books for families of people with mental illness.

Greist, John H., and James W. Jefferson. *Depression and Its Treatment: Help for the Nation's No. 1 Mental Problem.* Washington, DC: American Psychiatric Press, 1984. 128p. $7.95 (paperback). ISBN 0-88048-025-4.

> In nontechnical language, this book addresses basic issues about depression including its nature, its cause, and its treatment. This would be an excellent first book for a nonprofessional interested in becoming acquainted with facts about depressive illness.

Greist, John H., James W. Jefferson, and Isaac M. Marks. *Anxiety and Its Treatment: Help Is Available*. Washington, DC: American Psychiatric Press, 1986. 216p. $14.95. ISBN 0-88048-212-5.

> This book, written for the general public, describes different types of anxiety disorders and their pharmacologic and psychologic treatments. It offers suggestions about what a person with an anxiety disorder can do for him- or herself to improve the problem. Replete with case examples, this is a clearly written and useful guide for nonprofessionals.

Korpell, Herbert S. *How You Can Help: A Guide for Families of Psychiatric Hospital Patients*. Washington, DC: American Psychiatric Press, 1984. 156p. $15.95. ISBN 0-88048-016-5. $9.95 (paperback). ISBN 0-88048-026-2.

> *How You Can Help* is a useful guide for families of persons who may be psychiatrically hospitalized. The author, a psychiatrist, addresses issues of frequent concern to families such as: Who needs psychiatric hospitalization? How is a patient evaluated at a psychiatric hospital? What are psychiatric disorders? What sorts of treatments are provided in a psychiatric hospital? How can a family member be of assistance to the patient before, during, and after hospitalization?

Lewinsohn, Peter M., Ricardo F. Munoz, Mary Ann Youngren, and Antonette M. Zeiss. *Control Your Depression*. New York: Prentice-Hall, 1986. 241p. $9.95 (paperback). ISBN 0-13-171893-2.

> The senior author of this book is a leading figure in research and therapy for depression from a social learning theory point of view. The book reviews basic principles and techniques used to reduce symptoms of depression. For example, it contains step-by-step instructions for becoming more relaxed, increasing the frequency of pleasurable activities, reducing thoughts related to depression, and enhancing social skills. The volume includes copies of schedules, questionnaires, and checklists that may be utilized as part of a self-directed program to reduce depression.

Zane, Manuel D., and Harry Milt. *Your Phobia: Understanding Your Fears through Contextual Therapy*. Washington, DC: American Psychiatric Press, 1984. 304p. $15.95. ISBN 0-88048-008-4.

This volume is written by proponents of a contextual therapy approach to the treatment of phobias. The premise of contextual therapy is that confrontation with an object or situation about which the individual is phobic can eliminate the phobia. The authors review general issues on phobias, use many case examples, and outline specific efforts in which the phobic individual may engage to control phobic feelings.

MENTAL HEALTH AND AGING

Billig, Nathan. *To Be Old and Sad: Understanding Depression in the Elderly.* Lexington, MA: Lexington Books, 1987. 128p. $21.95. ISBN 0-669-12277-7. $8.95 (paper). ISBN 0-669-12279-3.

This is a book primarily written for nonprofessionals who want to learn more about depression in older adults. It is a clear summary of what is known about depression in late life, its treatment, its relationship with dementia, and its prognosis. The book would be especially useful for family members of older individuals with depression.

Butler, Robert N., and Myrna I. Lewis. *Aging and Mental Health.* Consumer's ed. St. Louis: Mosby, 1983. 386p. $8.95 (paper). ISBN 0-8016-1002-8.

This is an edition of the authors' book *Aging and Mental Health: Positive Psychosocial and Biomedical Approaches* that was rewritten for nonprofessionals (consumers). The book discusses the nature of aging, problems of older adults, and the evaluation, treatment, and prevention of late-life mental health problems.

Eisdorfer, Carl, and Donna Cohen. *The Loss of Self: A Family Resource for the Care of Alzheimer's Disease and Related Disorders.* New York: W. W. Norton, 1986. 381p. $19.95. ISBN 0-393-02263-3.

This book was written by two well-known geriatric mental health professionals who played a key role in initially alerting the professional community to the needs of dementia patients and their families. The authors draw on their extensive professional experience to discuss a variety of issues that would be of concern to family members of dementia patients. The book contains a useful appendix with suggestions for additional reading, a list of organizations concerned with aging, and information on legal and financial issues.

Hooyman, Nancy R., and Wendy Lustbader. *Taking Care: Supporting Older People and Their Families.* New York: Free Press. 1986. 320p. $24.95. ISBN 0-02-914900-2.

> This volume is a good blend of academic and practical approaches to the issues faced by family members caring for older adults. For the professional with an interest in this area, it is an orientation to many of the topics on caregiving currently being discussed and researched by gerontologists. For the nonprofessional, it contains useful information about social, psychological, service delivery, financial, and nursing home issues and practical suggestions on how to be a more effective and well-adjusted caregiver. The book also contains a fairly well selected group of suggestions for further reading.

Mace, Nancy L., and Peter V. Rabins. *The 36-Hour Day: A Family Guide to Caring for Persons with Alzheimer's Disease, Related Illnesses, and Memory Loss in Later Life.* Baltimore, MD: The Johns Hopkins University Press, 1982. 272p. $19.50. ISBN 0-8018-2659-4. $7.95 (paper). ISBN 0-8018-2660-8.

> This is *the* first serious treatment of the problems faced by people caring for dementia patients. It is an immensely practical book filled with information and suggestions on how to better cope with the myriad problems that emerge in caring for a dementia patient.

Powell, Lenore S., and Katie Courtice. *Alzheimer's Disease: A Guide for Families.* Reading, MA: Addison-Wesley, 1983. 288p. $8.95 (paperback). ISBN 0-201-06099-X.

> This volume is a resource for caregivers of dementia patients. It describes the characteristic problems associated with dementia and offers suggestions on how to best deal with them. An important focus of the volume is on the psychological and emotional difficulties experienced by caregivers (e.g., anger, depression, guilt, and confusion or ambivalence about options), and it also offers guidance on how to better cope with such difficulties. The book provides helpful suggestions on how the caregiver can better care for his or her own physical health.

Reisberg, Barry. *A Guide to Alzheimer's Disease: For Families, Spouses, and Friends*. New York: Free Press, 1981. 216p. $8.95 (paperback). ISBN 0-02-926370-0.

> This book was written by a psychiatrist who has played an important role in doing research on and providing services to patients with dementia. It is a well-documented and well-written discussion of Alzheimer's disease and other dementias; it also offers some guidance on the clinical management of this condition. Although the book is somewhat dated, it still provides a good treatment of the subject and is useful for both professionals and nonprofessionals.

Richards, Marty, Nancy Hooyman, Mary Hansen, Wendy Brandts, Kathy Smith-DiJulio, and Lynn Dahm. *Choosing a Nursing Home: A Guidebook for Families*. Seattle: University of Washington Press, 1985. 112p. $8.95 (paperback). ISBN 0-295-96221-6.

> This volume offers valuable information to older people considering entering a nursing home and their families. It orients the individual to the issues that need to be considered in choosing a nursing home, adjusting to nursing home life, and negotiating the bureaucratic, financial, and social service systems that are connected with nursing home placement. It also offers family members of nursing home residents practical advice on how to make visits satisfying and meaningful for both parties.

Pamphlets

> Some organizations have developed pamphlets for the general public on different topics in mental health and/or aging. A selected group of these pamphlets is reviewed below. The reader is urged, however, to contact the organizations that distribute these for a current list of pamphlets and other materials. New publications are often added, and supplies of existing materials are sometimes exhausted. Organizations also offer other materials that may not be reviewed here and that would be of interest to some. The addresses of organizations that produce these materials may be found in Chapter 5 in the section titled "National Resources." Unless otherwise indicated, single copies of the materials listed below are available free of charge.

The Alzheimer's Association

Alzheimer's Disease: An Overview. 1987. 10p. ED 211 Z.

> This pamphlet describes Alzheimer's disease, its symptoms, those most vulnerable to it, its diagnosis, possible causes, outcome, and available help. A brief glossary is included as well as three suggestions for further reading.

Alzheimer's Disease: Services You May Need. 1987. 10p. ED 210 Z.

> Health care, respite, long-term care, and support services that might be needed by people with dementia and their families are discussed. Places to look for services and three recommendations for further reading are included.

Assisting the Person with Alzheimer's. 1988. 23p. ED/303/Z.

> Practical suggestions on how family members may deal with a range of problematic behaviors evidenced by the dementia patient are discussed. Behaviors include forgetfulness, repetitiveness, difficulty with organization, disorientation, difficulty with calculations, changes in writing, inappropriate facial expressions, hoarding, and suspiciousness and paranoia. Three recommendations for further reading are included.

Caregiving at Home. 1987. 10p. ED 213 Z.

> The pamphlet discusses basic issues in caring for a person with dementia at home. It includes two recommendations for further reading.

Communicating with the Alzheimer Patient. 1988. 8p. ED 220 Z.

> This outlines basic issues in the often difficult process of trying to verbally (and nonverbally) communicate with a dementia patient.

Financial Services You May Need. 1988. 10p. ED 222 Z.

> This reviews basic issues in how to pay for health and related care for a person with dementia. One book and three brochures are suggested for further reading.

Home Care with the Alzheimer Patient. 1988. 27p. ED/302/Z.

> This booklet addresses common problems confronted by family members caring for dementia patients and offers concrete sug-

gestions on how to manage such problems. Four books are recommended for further reading.

If You Have Alzheimer's Disease: What You Should Know, What You Can Do. 1987. 8p. No identifying numbers.

> This is a unique pamphlet designed for the person with Alzheimer's disease. It addresses basic issues of concern including what the disease is, how it will affect the person's life, how to manage things on a day-by-day basis, and issues in planning for the future. The pamphlet frankly addresses the fact that Alzheimer's is a progressive disease that will affect a range of abilities, but it communicates the message that the patient can do a variety of things to meet the challenge of dementia.

Legal Considerations for Alzheimer's Disease. 1987. 10p. ED 208 Z.

> This publication describes basic legal issues that families of persons with dementia need to know. These include power of attorney, durable power of attorney, living trust, will, living will, conservatorship of property, and guardianship or conservatorship. Suggestions for ways to find legal help are offered. Two books are listed for further reading.

Memory and Aging. 1987. 4p. ED 207 Z.

> This brochure clarifies the difference between normal age-associated memory impairment and dementia. Two books for further reading are included.

American Psychiatric Association

Let's Talk Facts About: Anxiety Disorders. 1988. 8p.

> The nature of phobias, panic disorders, post-traumatic stress disorder, and obsessive-compulsive disorder is reviewed. Theories about their causes and existing treatments are briefly outlined. The pamphlet includes eleven items for further reading and two organizations that could be contacted for further information.

Let's Talk Facts About: Depression. 1988. 10p.

> Symptoms of depression, possible causes, and current treatments are outlined. Five books for further reading and four organizations that could be contacted for further information are included.

Let's Talk Facts About: Manic-Depressive Disorder. 1988. 8p.

> Symptoms of manic-depressive illness (bipolar disorder), theories about its cause, and existing treatments are briefly discussed. Six books are recommended for further reading and four mental health organizations are listed.

Let's Talk Facts About: Mental Health of the Elderly. 1988. 8p.

> General issues concerning mental health and older adults are discussed and problems of depression and dementia are highlighted. Eleven books on issues relating to mental health and the elderly are recommended and seven organizations concerned with mental health and/or aging are listed.

Let's Talk Facts About: Mental Illness: There Are a Lot of Troubled People. 1988. 12p.

> An overview of mental illnesses in U.S. society, recent advances in diagnosis and treatment of mental disorders, and a discussion of depression, anxiety, and schizophrenia are included.

Let's Talk Facts About: Obsessive-Compulsive Disorder. 1988. 8p.

> Symptoms of obsessive-compulsive disorder, theories about its causes, and current treatments are outlined. Four books for additional reading are listed and the address of a self-help group for people with obsessive-compulsive disorders is provided.

Let's Talk Facts About: Phobias. 1988. 8p.

> The nature of and treatments for agoraphobia, social phobia, and simple phobias are reviewed. A bibliography of eleven books is included and names and addresses of four mental health–related organizations are listed.

Let's Talk Facts About: Schizophrenia. 1988. 10p.

> Symptoms of schizophrenia, its prevalence, theories about its causes, and treatments are covered. Six books for additional reading are included along with the names of four mental health–associated organizations.

Let's Talk Facts About: Substance Abuse. 1988. 27p.

> Problems with alcohol and drug use are discussed. The nature of problems with alcohol and drugs, usual difficulties associated with alcohol and drug use, and possible treatments for commonly

used drugs are outlined. Substances addressed include alcohol, marijuana, cocaine, opiates, hallucinogens, inhalants, sedative-hypnotics, and nicotine. Twenty-one books and pamphlets on alcohol and drug use are listed along with names, addresses, and phone numbers of organizations that could be of assistance to persons seeking information or help for alcohol and drug use.

National Alliance for the Mentally Ill

Depressive Illness: Now You Can Learn How To Help. 6p.

This pamphlet provides a brief outline of information about depressive illness and the Depressive Illness Project of the National Alliance for the Mentally Ill (NAMI)—an effort to disseminate information about depressive illness. Three organizations are listed for further information on depression.

Mental Illness Is Everybody's Business. 6p.

This defines mental illness, schizophrenia, and affective disorders and discusses their possible causes and treatments. It suggests ways that people may affirmatively act for those who have mental illness and includes six recommended readings.

Papolos, Demitri. *Mood Disorders: Depression and Manic Depression.* 15p.

Using a question-and-answer format, basic issues about depression and manic depression are discussed, including the nature of these disorders, treatments, and prognosis. This is a particularly well written pamphlet.

What Is Schizophrenia? 8p.

This briefly describes what schizophrenia is, what it is not, how it is treated, and the role of the family in helping the patient.

National Institute on Aging

Age Pages. Rev. 1985. 98p. U.S. Government Printing Office: 1986-496-399.

This is a compilation of fact sheets called *Age Pages,* which are published by the National Institute on Aging. They cover a range of topics, most having to do with physical health in later life. An almost complete set of *Age Pages* is contained in the above publication (some *Age Pages* appeared after 1985, when existing pages were bound). Fact sheets relevant to mental health and aging are described below. Fact sheets on single topics may be requested in lieu of the bound set.

Age Page: Aging and Alcohol Abuse. 3p.

This discusses the problem of alcohol abuse in older adults, physical effects of alcohol, the effects of other drugs combined with alcohol, and how to get help for alcohol problems. Three organizations are listed for further information.

Age Page: Safe Use of Medicines in Older People. 2p.

This offers general guidelines for older adults in taking prescribed and over-the-counter medications. Two additional booklets on this topic are listed.

Age Page: Safe Use of Tranquilizers. 1989. 2p. U.S. Government Printing Office: 1989-242-787/00001.

The problems associated with use of tranquilizing medications are reviewed and general guidelines are given for their safe use. Four organizations are listed that may be contacted for further information.

Age Page: Senility: Myth or Madness? 3p.

This *Age Page* provides a brief overview of issues in the diagnosis, treatment, and prevention of dementia.

Age Page: When You Need a Nursing Home. 1986. 4p. U.S. Government Printing Office: 1986-491-280/40003.

Options for long-term care, how to choose a nursing home, and how to make a smooth transition to a nursing home are discussed. Three organizations that may be contacted for further information are listed and one booklet is recommended for additional reading.

Age Page: Who's Who in Health Care. 5p.

Different kinds of medical and mental health care providers are listed with the kind of training they have received and the scope of services they typically provide.

Alzheimer's Disease Research Center Program List. 2p.

> This is a periodically updated list of Alzheimer's Disease Research Center programs funded by the National Institute on Aging to investigate the causes of dementia and its treatment. A current listing of Alzheimer's Disease Research Centers is provided in Chapter 5 in the section titled "State and Local Resources."

Differential Diagnosis of Dementing Diseases: National Institutes of Health Consensus Development Conference Statement. 1987. 9p. U.S. Government Printing Office: 1987-181-196/6112B.

> This is a statement of general agreement among leading scientists on the definition of dementia, its evaluation, and priorities for further research in this area. This consensus statement contains important information for mental health professionals who diagnose and/or treat persons with dementia.

Progress Report on Alzheimer's Disease, Volume II. 1984. 27p. NIH Publication No. 84-2500.

> This pamphlet examines research efforts to understand the cause, mechanisms, and diagnosis of Alzheimer's disease and efforts to help families of afflicted individuals.

Q&A: Alzheimer's Disease. 1981. 12p. NIH Publication No. 81-1646.

> This publication examines the symptoms of Alzheimer's disease; its diagnosis, cause, and possible treatment; and research efforts to address it. A glossary is included.

National Institute of Mental Health

Bipolar Disorder: Manic-Depressive Illness. 1989. 6p. DHHS Publication No. (ADM) 89-1609.

> This briefly outlines the symptoms of and treatments for bipolar disorder. The pamphlet also includes a list of five organizations that may be contacted for further information.

A Consumer's Guide to Mental Health Services. Rev. 1987. 28p. DHHS Publication No. (ADM) 87-214.

> This pamphlet is an orientation to basic issues in the nature and treatment of different kinds of mental illness. It also defines the

kinds of services provided by different types of mental health professionals. The pamphlet provide names and addresses of 22 different organizations that may offer information on mental health issues.

Depression: What You Need To Know. 1987. 9p. DHHS Publication No. (ADM) 87-1543.

This pamphlet defines depression and mania, their possible causes, available treatments, side effects of antidepressants, general advice for people with depressive disorders, and how family and friends can help depressed persons.

Depressive Disorders: Treatments Bring New Hope. 1986. 25p. DHHS Publication No. (ADM) 86-1491.

The publication discusses what depression is, its possible causes, the risk of suicide, available treatments, the prevalence of depression in different age groups, how to be of assistance to a depressed person, and how to locate mental health services.

Fact Sheet: Depression in the Elderly. 1989. 4p.

The fact sheet defines depression and describes ways to recognize its presence, when and where to seek treatment, and the prognosis of the illness.

Helpful Facts about Depressive Disorders. 1989. 8p. DHHS Publication No. (ADM) 89-1536.

This pamphlet offers a brief outline of basic issues in the definition, nature, and treatment of mania and depression.

Information on Lithium. 1981. 7p. DHHS Publication No. (ADM) 81-1078.

This describes the psychotropic medication lithium and the purposes for which it is prescribed. The pamphlet includes a checklist of issues about which the person taking lithium should be aware and a list of six additional publications about lithium.

Plain Talk about Aging. Rep. 1985. 4p. DHHS Publication No. (ADM) 85-1266.

This is a brief outline of issues that bear on emotional and social adjustment to aging.

Plain Talk about Mutual Help Groups. Rep. 1983. 4p. DHHS
Publication No. (ADM) 83-1138.

> Mutual help (also called self-help or mutual aid) groups are dis-
> cussed. Their purpose, their modes of operation, their relation-
> ship with professionals, and how to locate them are reviewed. Ad-
> dresses and phone numbers of 32 mutual help groups are listed.

Schizophrenia: Questions and Answers. 1986. 25p. DHHS Publication
No. (ADM) 86-1457.

> The pamphlet address five questions commonly asked about schizo-
> phrenia: What is it? What is the cause of it? What treatments are
> available? How can other persons be of assistance to the individ-
> ual with schizophrenia? What is the prognosis for this illness?

Useful Information On . . . Alzheimer's Disease. 1987. 14p. DHHS
Publication No. (OM) 87-4025.

> This is an overview of the nature, possible causes, evaluation,
> and treatments of Alzheimer's disease.

Useful Information On . . . Medications for Mental Illness. 1987. 27p.
DHHS Publication No. (ADM) 87-1509.

> This pamphlet provides basic information on medications that
> are used to treat anxiety, depression, bipolar disorder, and
> schizophrenia. It briefly reviews special considerations in pre-
> scribing psychotropic drugs in certain populations, including the
> elderly, and has an alphabetical listing of psychotropic medica-
> tions by both generic and trade name. (Note: This listing of
> medications by generic and trade names is reproduced in Ap-
> pendix A of this book.)

Useful Information On . . . Phobias and Panic. Rep. 1987. 39p. DHHS
Publication No. (ADM) 87-1472.

> Types of phobias and panic disorders, their possible causes and
> treatments, and prognosis are discussed. A list of 12 publications
> for further reading on this topic is included.

Useful Information On . . . Suicide. 1986. 28p. DHHS Publication
No. (ADM) 86-1489.

> This pamphlet offers a historical overview of suicide and dis-
> cusses its risk factors, warning signs, treatment, and prevention.

Six organizations that may be contacted for further information are listed; an outline of general places to find mental health resources is provided; and five recommendations for further reading are included.

National Mental Health Association

Schizophrenia. 1986. 6p.

Symptoms of and treatment for schizophrenia are outlined.

Stigma: A Lack of Awareness and Understanding. 1987. 8p. PU1907-8/87-10K.

This addresses basic misconceptions about mental illness. It also discusses different kinds of mental illness including depression, manic depression (bipolar disorder), schizophrenia, anxiety disorders, and eating disorders.

Stress: A Fact of Life. 1988. 8p. PU1908-7/88-20K.

This publication discusses the nature and effect of everyday stress on the individual and offers suggestions on how to better manage stress. General recommendations are included on where to find help for stress-related problems.

Films and Videocassettes

Although there are very few audiovisual materials on mental health and aging, some materials on Alzheimer's disease and issues in caring for physically or cognitively impaired older persons have been produced in recent years. The following is a summary of some of the better audiovisual materials on dementia, caregiving, and a few other aspects of mental health in later life.

Alcohol, Drugs, and Seniors: Tarnished Dreams
Type: 1/2" and 3/4" color video; 16mm color film
Length: 23 min.
Date: 1987
Cost: Purchase $370 (video), $495 (film); rental $75 (film)

Source: AIMS Media
6901 Woodley Avenue
Van Nuys, CA 91406-4878

This film describes the problems of alcohol and drug abuse in older adults. It is narrated by actor John Austin and uses four case vignettes. Difficulties in the recognition of these problems in older adults, the consequences of drug abuse and addiction, and the means by which professionals may treat the conditions are discussed. This film would be of interest to older persons and their families.

Caring: Families Coping with Alzheimer's Disease
Type: 1/2" and 3/4" color video
Length: 30 min.
Date: 1982
Cost: Not for sale; contact Alzheimer's Association for loan information
Source: Local chapter of the Alzheimer's Association; for location of nearest chapter, contact:
The Alzheimer's Association
70 East Lake Street, Suite 600
Chicago, IL 60601
(800) 621-0379; in Illinois (800) 572-6037

This video provides clearly presented factual information about dementia and highlights the problems faced by three families of older people with dementing illness. The production also illustrates various means by which family members cope with their difficulties. The film was developed for use by local chapters of the Alzheimer's Association and would be particularly valuable for families of persons with dementia.

Caring . . . Sharing: The Alzheimer's Caregiver
Type: 1/2" and 3/4" color video
Length: 30 min.
Date: 1987
Cost: Purchase $250 (1/2"), $265 (3/4"); no rental
Source: Hal Kirn and Associates
2122 Wallace Street
Philadelphia, PA 19130

The format of this video is a discussion among members of a support group for dementia caregivers. The strains of caregiving, the demands of problem-solving the complex difficulties that often exist, the caregiver's experience of strong emotions, and the need for support from others are explored. People caring for dementia patients are the best audience for this video.

The Case of John R.: Depression among Older Persons

Type: 1/2" and 3/4" color video
Length: 59 min.
Date: 1987
Cost: Purchase $230, rental $30
Source: Growing Edge Productions
           P.O. Box 6296
           Evanston, IL 60202

This is a videotape of a clinical case conference among three human service providers regarding a 73-year-old man who is depressed. The discussants bring different theoretical approaches to the understanding of the nature and treatment of John R.'s depression.

Coping and Home Safety Tips for Caregivers of the Elderly

Type: 1/2" color video
Length: 17 min.
Date: 1987
Cost: Purchase $89.95, rental $10
Source: Jefferson Area Board for Aging
           423 Lexington Avenue
           Charlottesville, VA 22901

The purpose of this video, which is accompanied by a training manual, is to teach family members caring for physically or cognitively impaired older adults how to better manage the practical issues involved in caregiving. The video includes, for example, recommendations on how to help the older person eat, toilet, dress, and safely ambulate. This video would be most useful for family caregivers.

Four Lives: A Portrait of Manic Depression

Type: 1/2" and 3/4" color video; 16mm color film
Length: 60 min.
Date: 1987

Cost: Purchase $430 (video), $700 (film); rental $75 per day or
           $150 per week (video only)
Source: Fanlight Productions
           47 Halifax Street
           Boston, MA 02130

Making extensive use of interviews, the film discusses the nature,
cause, consequences, and treatments of bipolar disorder (manic-
depressive illness). Although the film does not not address the
unique problems of older adults with this disorder, it is a useful
general discussion of bipolar illness. This film would be of interest to professionals and nonprofessionals unfamiliar with this
mental health problem.

In Care of: Families and Their Elders
Type: 1/2" and 3/4" color video
Length: 55 min.
Date: 1988
Cost: Purchase $295 (1/2"), $345 (3/4"); rental $50
Source: The Brookdale Center on Aging of Hunter College
           425 East 25th Street
           New York, NY 10010

In this video, four families tell of their experiences in caring for
an older person with a physical (e.g., blindness or stroke) or
mental (e.g., cognitive impairment) disability. In the first part of
the video the burdens as well as the satisfactions of caregiving are
conveyed in a thoughtful and sensitive way. In the second part of
this presentation, different kinds of formal services sometimes
available to family caregivers are described. The video is hosted
by Hugh Downs and would be of interest to family members
caring for impaired relatives and to professionals unfamiliar
with these issues.

Managing with Alzheimer's Disease
Type: 1/2" and 3/4" color video
Length: 30 min.
Date: 1983
Cost: Purchase $195, rental $45
Source: Media Technology Department
           Good Samaritan Hospital
           1015 N.W. 22nd
           Portland, OR 97210

This video outlines practical steps that can be taken by families of people with dementia to deal with care-related problems. For example, suggestions are offered on how to deal with sleep, eating, personal care, safety, and communication difficulties. The video is best suited for family members of persons newly diagnosed with dementia. Professionals unfamiliar with the problems faced by families caring for dementia patients at home would also find the video useful.

Medication and Dementia

Type:	1/2″ and 3/4″ color video
Length:	20 min.
Date:	1987
Cost:	Purchase $300, rental $100
Source:	Video Services
	Department of Physical Therapy, School of Medicine
	University of Maryland
	32 South Greene Street
	Baltimore, MD 21201

The format of this film is a discussion between a pharmacist and an expert on geriatric pharmacology about the effects of medication on older adults. The main emphasis in the video is on how medications may cause reversible cognitive impairment or exacerbate symptoms in persons with irreversible dementia. The video underscores the need for vigilance and caution in prescribing drugs for older adults. The video would be of use to professionals, paraprofessionals, older people, and family members.

There Were Times, Dear

Type:	1/2″ color video; 16mm color film
Length:	60 min.
Date:	1985
Cost:	Purchase $250 (video), $895 (film); rental $50 (video), $85 (film); also available free to groups that use the film to fundraise for Alzheimer's research or support groups
Source:	Direct Cinema
	P.O. Box 69589
	Los Angeles, CA 90069

Sandoz Pharmaceutical Corporation
Route 10
East Hanover, NJ 07936

This film follows a man diagnosed with Alzheimer's disease and his family for five years. The nature, diagnosis, and prognosis of Alzheimer's disease are discussed. The practical and emotional problems faced by families of people with this condition are also examined. This film would be of interest to both professionals and a general audience. A discussion guide accompanies the video and film.

Understanding and Coping with Dementia

Type: 1/2″ and 3/4″ (set of three color videos)
Length: 32 min. each
Date: 1985
Cost: Purchase $60 each video, no rental
Source: Suncoast Gerontology Center
          University of South Florida Medical Center
          Box 50, 12901 North 30th Street
          Tampa, FL 33612

In these videos the topic of dementia is explored through interviews of people with dementia and their families. Part One of the set of three videos examines recognition and diagnosis of dementia; Part Two discusses the management of cognitive disorders; and Part Three examines the course of dementia and its outcome. These videos would be of interest to professionals and to some general audiences.

We're Not Alone

Type: 1/2″ color video
Length: 28 min.
Date: 1987
Cost: Purchase $175 (nonprofit), $500 (profit); no rental; $50 preview fee applied toward purchase
Source: Bell Direct, Inc.
          7 Nowell Farme Road
          Carlisle, MA 01741

This video is part of a package of materials that includes a 43-minute audiocassette describing "A Caregiver's Bill of Rights" and an "Information and Action Manual." Narrated by Colleen

Dewhurst, the video discusses problems faced by individuals caring for impaired older family members and possible solutions to those problems. The video is meant to raise the viewer's level of awareness about caregiving issues and is appropriate for businesspeople and social service workers.

Glossary

adjustment disorder Poor adaptation to a clearly identifiable life stressor or stressors. This condition is usually accompanied by symptoms of emotional distress such as depression or anxiety.

agoraphobia Fearfulness about being in a situation from which one might not escape easily.

Alzheimer's disease An organic brain disorder characterized by progressive loss of cognitive abilities. The cause or causes of Alzheimer's disease are currently unknown.

anticholinergic side effects In the mental health field, refers to side effects (such as dry mouth, blurry vision, or constipation) of certain psychiatric medications because of their effects on the cholinergic nervous system.

antidepressants Medications used in the treatment of certain kinds of depression.

anxiety Feelings of tension or uneasiness that may accompany a normal response to life circumstances or that may be severe or disabling, as those that often accompany certain anxiety disorders.

barbiturates Prior to the introduction of benzodiazepines, a type of medication that was frequently used to treat severe anxiety disorders.

behaviorism A psychological theory and approach to mental health treatment that posits that people's behavior is strongly influenced by the rewards, lack of rewards, or punishments that precede or follow behavior.

bereavement   Normal feelings of sadness and desolation following the death of person to whom an individual was emotionally attached.

beta-blockers   An abbreviation for beta-adrenergic blocking agents. Primarily used in the treatment of certain medical conditions but also prescribed for some anxiety disorders.

bipolar disorder   A condition in which individuals usually experience episodes of mania and depression. Formerly called manic depression.

board and care facilities   A type of nursing home that provides room and board and sometimes offers social and recreational activities. Chronically mentally ill persons sometimes live in such residences.

catecholamine hypothesis   A theory that three brain substances, norepinephrine, dopamine, and serotonin, play a major role in regulation of mood.

clinical depression   A general reference to feelings of depression and other symptoms that are so severe or long-lasting as to warrant help from a mental health professional.

cognitive therapy   An approach to mental health practice based on the premise that a critical determinant of emotional states is the way an individual thinks about himself/herself, his/her experiences, and the future.

compulsions   Actions typically performed in response to an obsessional idea.

couple psychotherapy   A psychotherapeutic approach in which two individuals meet with a mental health professional to try to change common problems. The most frequent participants in couple psychotherapy are people with marital problems.

Creutzfeldt-Jakob disease   A rare form of dementia with symptoms similar to Alzheimer's disease that may be virally transmitted.

CT scan   Abbreviation for computerized axial transverse tomography scan in which multiple X-ray pictures are taken of the brain.

cyclothymia   A less severe form of bipolar disorder in which an individual has ongoing disturbances of mood with periods of hypomania and symptoms of depression.

delirium   An organic mental syndrome that involves problems with maintaining and shifting attention, logical thinking, speech, and other difficulties.

delusional disorder   A mental disorder in which there is the persistent presence of a delusion, usually of a persecutory nature.

delusions   Beliefs held by an individual that reflect a significant distortion of reality.

dementia   An organic mental syndrome in which deficits in short-term and long-term memory are evident. It is often accompanied by difficulties in thinking and judgment, personality changes, and other cognitive problems.

depression   An emotional state typically characterized by feelings of being sad, downhearted, blue, or similar descriptors.

The Diagnostic and Statistical Manual of Mental Disorders (DSM-III-R)   A manual devised by the American Psychiatric Association that contains specific rules for making a diagnosis of currently recognized mental disorders. The most recent version of the manual is a revision of the third edition.

dysthymia   A long-standing mood disorder characterized by feelings of depression and other symptoms that are usually less severe than those associated with major depression.

electrocardiogram (EKG)   A machine that measures different aspects of heart activity.

electroconvulsive therapy (ECT)   A procedure most commonly used in the treatment of some serious depressions, in which an electric current is passed through an individual's brain to induce a brief seizure. One theory is that seizure activity changes the balance of brain chemicals in a way that improves the individual's condition.

electroencephalogram (EEG)   A machine that measures electrical activity in the brain.

extrapyramidal side effects   A range of possible side effects of neuroleptic medications (for example, muscle spasms, restlessness, lack of energy).

family psychotherapy   A psychotherapeutic method in which some or all members of a family take part in a treatment designed to identify and remedy maladaptive patterns of interacting within the family.

general paresis   A dementia caused by neurosyphilis, a sexually transmitted bacterial infection.

generalized anxiety disorder   A condition in which an individual is prone to excessive worry and anxiety.

group psychotherapy   A type of psychotherapy in which the power of the social group is used to effect psychological and social change in the individual. Groups are often composed of persons sharing the same type of problems.

hallucinations   False sensory perceptions that typically involve an individual hearing or seeing things that others do not.

hypertensive crisis   A significant increase in blood pressure that may result when a person taking MAO-inhibitor antidepressant medication consumes certain foods (such as aged cheeses) that contain tyramine. A hypertensive crisis increases risk of stroke.

hypomania   A less severe form of a manic episode.

kuru   A virally transmitted type of dementia found in New Guinea.

late paraphrenia   A term coined by British psychiatrist Sir Martin Roth to describe schizophrenia-like symptoms appearing for the first time in late life.

learning theory A psychological theory that posits that emotional responses are learned like any other behavior.

lithium A medication most frequently prescribed for the treatment of bipolar disorder.

long-term care Refers to a variety of institutional living arrangements for persons who are unable to live within the community due to physical or mental disabilities. These facilities range from "board and care" homes, in which only room and board are provided, to skilled nursing facilities, in which 24-hour medical care and supervision are provided.

major depression A mental disorder characterized by depressed mood and changes in behavior, thinking, and physiological processes such as sleep and appetite.

manic episode A specific period in which an individual's mood is characteristically elevated, expansive, or irritable. A manic episode is also accompanied by other symptoms.

mental status test A brief series of questions from which a mental health professional can make a general determination of the presence of cognitive impairment.

monoamine oxidase (MAO) A chemical substance believed to be involved in the deactivation of norepinephrine, a neurotransmitter hypothesized to play an important role in the regulation of mood.

monoamine oxidase inhibitor (MAO-I) A type of antidepressant medication thought to reduce the activity of MAO, a substance that breaks down norepinephrine.

mood disorder A disturbance of normal emotional states, usually evidenced in depression or mania, that typically requires treatment from a mental health professional.

MRI scan Abbreviation for magnetic resonance imaging, a machine that precisely measures structures in the brain using a magnetic field.

multi-infarct dementia   A condition in which there is a progressive loss of cognitive abilities through a series of small strokes caused by blockages of arteries to the brain.

neuroleptic medications   A type of psychiatric medication often used in the treatment of psychotic symptoms. Neuroleptic medications are part of a class of drugs call major tranquilizers.

neurotransmitters   Chemical substances in the brain involved in the communication of information across specialized brain cells called neurons.

nonprogressive dementias   Dementing conditions usually caused by brain injuries that typically impair select cognitive abilities. The most common type of nonprogressive dementias result from strokes, head trauma, and aneurysms.

normal pressure hydrocephalus   A condition caused by obstruction of the movement of cerebrospinal fluid that results in dementia. If the condition is corrected there may be considerable reduction in dementia symptoms.

obsessions   Images, thoughts, or ideas that persistently return and may be regarded by the individual as senseless.

obsessive-compulsive disorder   A condition in which the individual has recurring obsessions or compulsions that are severe enough to interfere with emotional, interpersonal, or occupational functioning.

orthostatic hypotension   A sudden drop in blood pressure most likely to occur when an individual either sits up or stands up quickly. Possibly a side effect of tricyclic antidepressant medications.

panic disorder   A condition in which an individual has recurrent episodes of extreme fear and discomfort that usually last a few minutes.

Parkinson's disease   A neurological disorder characterized by difficulties in moving, muscular rigidity, shaking, and often cognitive deficits.

PET scan   Abbreviation for positron emission tomography, an instrument that measures the metabolic activity of the brain.

pharmacokinetics   The physical process by which drugs enter the system, are dispersed throughout the body, and then are eliminated.

Pick's disease   A rare dementing disorder with symptoms similar to Alzheimer's disease but whose onset is usually between the ages of 40 and 60.

prevalence   Number of cases of a disease during a specified period of time.

prodromal   The early symptoms of an illness.

pseudodementia   Refers to cognitive changes that, on successful treatment of a psychiatric problem like depression, are no longer evident. Also called reversible dementia caused by depression.

psychiatric diagnosis   The general characterization of a set of problems experienced by an individual that are defined by established rules.

psychoactive substance abuse   The use of psychoactive substances (such as alcohol or drugs) that may cause a variety of social, psychological, occupational, or health-related problems that are not as severe as those resulting from psychoactive substance dependence.

psychoactive substance dependence   The use of psychoactive substances (such as alcohol or drugs) that may cause several of a variety of social, psychological, occupational, and health-related problems. Symptoms of substance withdrawal or tolerance may exist.

psychoanalysis   A body of theory and mental health practice, originally developed by Sigmund Freud, that places emphasis on early childhood experiences, particularly those involving sex or aggression, as critical determinants of later psychological development.

psychodynamic therapy   A treatment approach in which the realization and emotional "working through" of underlying conflicts, particularly those from early childhood, are thought to improve the individual's mental health.

psychomotor agitation   Clearly observable increases in an individual's level of physical activity, such as pacing or hand-wringing. Psychomotor agitation sometimes accompanies certain psychiatric disorders.

psychomotor retardation   Clearly observable decreases in an individual's level of physical activity, such as slowness of eye-blinking or movement.

psychopharmacology   The study of drug treatments for people with psychiatric difficulties.

psychotherapy   The application of different psychological techniques by a mental health professional to change certain ways of feeling, thinking, or behaving that are experienced by the individual as unpleasant or undesirable.

psychotic   Refers to serious impairment in the ability to accurately perceive reality, such as evidenced in delusions and hallucinations.

psychotropic medications   Drugs used in the treatment of certain mental disorders.

schizophrenia   A brain disorder characterized by a variety of psychotic and nonpsychotic symptoms the onset of which is almost always in early life.

simple phobia   An ongoing fear of a specific object or situation such as animals, heights, closed spaces, blood, or traveling by air.

social phobia   An ongoing fear of being scrutinized, embarrassed, or humiliated by others while engaging in a particular behavior(s).

sociology   The study of the explicit and implicit rules that govern society.

somatic treatment   In mental health, treatment for mental disorders including medications or electroconvulsive therapy. The term is sometimes used to distinguish these treatments from psychological intervention such as psychotherapy.

stress   Feelings brought on by situations that tax or exceed an individual's perceived ability to manage them.

supportive psychotherapy   General efforts by a mental health professional to provide support, encouragement, and acceptance to a patient.

symptom   A specific manifestation of a disease or disorder.

syndrome   A specific group of mental or physical symptoms that usually occur together and are associated with a particular condition.

tardive dyskinesia   Involuntary muscle movements that are sometimes caused by exposure to neuroleptics.

therapeutic nihilism   An attitude on the part of some health professionals that little can be done for the mental health problems of many older adults (or other groups) because of the age of the patient and/or the severity of the problems.

thought disorder   Disturbances in the way that the individual's thinking processes are organized, such as the lack of logical associations between ideas. Also called conceptual disorganization.

tricyclic antidepressants   A type of antidepressant thought to increase the amount of norepinephrine in the brain. Depletion of norepinephrine is hypothesized to play a critical role in mood disorders.

vegetative symptoms   In the mental health field, refers to physiological changes such as sleep and appetite disturbance that are part of a particular psychiatric syndrome.

Appendixes

Appendix A

Alphabetic Listing of Psychotropic Medications by Generic and Trade Names

To find the section of the text that describes the drug you or a friend or family member is taking, find either the generic (chemical) name and look it up on the first list, or the trade name and look it up on the second list. If you do not find the name of the drug on the label, ask your doctor or pharmacist for it. (Note: some drugs, such as amitriptyline and chlordiazepoxide, are marketed under numerous trade names, not all of which can be mentioned in a brief [list] such as this. If your drug's trade name does not appear in this list, look it up by its generic name or ask your doctor or pharmacist for more information.)

Alphabetic Listing of Medications by Generic Name

GENERIC NAME	TRADE NAME	TYPE OF DRUG
acetophenazine	Tindal	antipsychotic
alprazolam	Xanax	antianxiety
amitriptyline	Amitid Amitril Elavil Endep	antidepressant
amoxapine	Ascendin	antidepressant
butaperazine	Repoise	antipsychotic
carbamazepine	Tegretol	antimanic
carphenazine	Proketazine	antipsychotic
chlordiazepoxide	Librax Libritabs Librium	antianxiety
chlorpromazine	Thorazine	antipsychotic
chlorprothixene	Taractan	antipsychotic
clorazepate	Azene Tranxene	antianxiety

Medications by Generic Name (continued)

GENERIC NAME	TRADE NAME	TYPE OF DRUG
desipramine	Norpramin Pertofrane	antidepressant
dextroamphetamine	Dexedrine	stimulant
diazepam✓	Valium ✓	antianxiety
doxepin	Adapin Sinequan	antidepressant
fluphenazine	Permitil Prolixin	antipsychotic
haloperidol	Haldol	antipsychotic
halazepam ✓	Paxipam ✓	antianxiety
imipramine	Imavate Janimine Presamine Tofranil	antidepressant
isocarboxazid	Marplan	antidepressant
lithium carbonate	Eskalith Lithane Lithobid	antimanic
lithium citrate	Cibalith-S	antimanic
lorazepam ✓	Ativan ✓	antianxiety
loxapine	Daxolin Loxitane	antipsychotic
maprotiline	Ludiomil	antidepressant
mesoridazine	Serentil	antipsychotic
methylphenidate	Ritalin	stimulant
molindone	Lidone Moban	antipsychotic
nortriptyline	Aventyl Pamelor	antidepressant
oxazepam ✓	Serax ✓	antianxiety
perphenazine	Trilafon	antipsychotic
phenelzine	Nardil	antidepressant
piperacetazine	Quide	antipsychotic
prazepam ✓	Centrax ✓ Vestran ✓	antianxiety
prochlorperazine	Compazine	antipsychotic
protriptyline	Vivactil	antidepressant
thioridazine	Mellaril	antipsychotic
thiothixene	Navane	antipsychotic
tranylcypromine	Parnate	antidepressant
trazodone	Desyrel	antidepressant

Medications by Generic Name   (continued)

GENERIC NAME	TRADE NAME	TYPE OF DRUG
trifluoperazine	Stelazine	antipsychotic
triflupromazine	Vesprin	antipsychotic

Alphabetic Listing of Medications by Trade Name

TRADE NAME	GENERIC NAME	TYPE OF DRUG
Adapin	doxepin	antidepressant
Amitid	amitriptyline	antidepressant
Amitril	amitriptyline	antidepressant
Ascendin	amoxapine	antidepressant
Ativan	lorazepam	antianxiety
Aventyl	nortriptyline	antidepressant
Azene	clorazepate	antianxiety
Centrax	prazepam	antianxiety
Cibalith-S	lithium citrate	antimanic
Compazine	prochlorperazine	antipsychotic
Daxolin	loxapine	antipsychotic
Desyrel	trazodone	antidepressant
Dexedrine	dextroamphetamine	stimulant
Elavil	amitriptyline	antidepressant
Endep	amitriptyline	antidepressant
Eskalith	lithium carbonate	antimanic
Haldol	haloperidol	antipsychotic
Imavate	imipramine	antidepressant
Janimine	imipramine	antidepressant
Librax	chlordiazepoxide	antianxiety
Libritabs	chlordiazepoxide	antianxiety
Librium	chlordiazepoxide	antianxiety
Lidone	molindone	antipsychotic
Lithane	lithium carbonate	antimanic
Lithobid	lithium carbonate	antimanic
Loxitane	loxapine	antipsychotic
Ludiomil	maprotiline	antidepressant
Marplan	isocarboxazid	antidepressant
Mellaril	thioridazine	antipsychotic
Moban	molindone	antipsychotic
Nardil	phenelzine	antidepressant
Navane	thiothixene	antipsychotic
Norpramin	desipramine	antidepressant
Pamelor	nortriptyline	antidepressant
Parnate	tranylcypromine	antidepressant
Paxipam	halazepam	antianxiety
Permitil	fluphenazine	antipsychotic
Pertofrane	desipramine	antidepressant
Presamine	imipramine	antidepressant
Proketazine	carphenazine	antipsychotic

Medications by Trade Name   (continued)

TRADE NAME	GENERIC NAME	TYPE OF DRUG
Prolixin	fluphenazine	antipsychotic
Quide	piperacetazine	antipsychotic
Repoise	butaperazine	antipsychotic
Ritalin	methylphenidate	stimulant
Serax	oxazepam	antianxiety
Serentil	mesoridazine	antipsychotic
Sinequan	doxepin	antidepressant
Stelazine	trifluoperazine	antipsychotic
Taractan	chlorprothixene	antipsychotic
Tegretol	carbamazepine	antimanic
Thorazine	chlorpromazine	antipsychotic
Tindal	acetophenazine	antipsychotic
Tofranil	imipramine	antidepressant
Tranxene	clorazepate	antianxiety
Trilafon	perphenazine	antipsychotic
Valium	diazepam	antianxiety
Vesprin	trifluopromazine	antipsychotic
Vestran	prazepam	antianxiety
Vivactil	protriptyline	antidepressant
Xanax	alprazolam	antianxiety

Reprinted from: The National Institute of Mental Health. *Useful Information On: Medications for Mental Illness.* 1987. DHHS Pub. No. (ADM) 87–1509.

Appendix B

Summary of Criteria for *DSM-III-R* Disorders

Diagnostic criteria for Major Depressive Episode

Note: A "Major Depressive Syndrome" is defined as criterion A below.

A. At least five of the following symptoms have been present during the same two-week period and represent a change from previous functioning; at least one of the symptoms is either (1) depressed mood, or (2) loss of interest or pleasure. (Do not include symptoms that are clearly due to a physical condition, mood-incongruent delusions or hallucinations, incoherence, or marked loosening of associations.)

    (1) depressed mood (or can be irritable mood in children and adolescents) most of the day, nearly every day, as indicated either by subjective account or observation by others

    (2) markedly diminished interest or pleasure in all, or almost all, activities most of the day, nearly every day (as indicated either by subjective account or observation by others of apathy most of the time)

    (3) significant weight loss or weight gain when not dieting (e.g., more than 5% of body weight in a month), or decrease or increase in appetite nearly every day (in children, consider failure to make expected weight gains)

    (4) insomnia or hypersomnia nearly every day

    (5) psychomotor agitation or retardation nearly every day (observable by others, not merely subjective feelings of restlessness or being slowed down)

    (6) fatigue or loss of energy nearly every day

    (7) feelings of worthlessness or excessive or inappropriate guilt (which may be delusional) nearly every day (not merely self-reproach or guilt about being sick)

    (8) diminished ability to think or concentrate, or indecisiveness, nearly every day (either by subjective account or as observed by others)

(9) recurrent thoughts of death (not just fear of dying), recurrent suicidal ideation without a specific plan, or a suicide attempt or a specific plan for committing suicide

B. (1) It cannot be established that an organic factor initiated and maintained the disturbance

    (2) The disturbance is not a normal reaction to the death of a loved one (Uncomplicated Bereavement)

    Note: Morbid preoccupation with worthlessness, suicidal ideation, marked functional impairment or psychomotor retardation, or prolonged duration suggest bereavement complicated by Major Depression.

C. At no time during the disturbance have there been delusions or hallucinations for as long as two weeks in the absence of prominent mood symptoms (i.e., before the mood symptoms developed or after they have remitted).

D. Not superimposed on Schizophrenia, Schizophreniform Disorder, Delusional Disorder, or Psychotic Disorder NOS.

Major Depressive Episode codes: Criteria for severity of current state of Bipolar Disorder, Depressed, or Major Depression:

1-Mild: Few, if any, symptoms in excess of those required to make the diagnosis, **and** symptoms result in only minor impairment in occupational functioning or in usual social activities or relationships with others.

2-Moderate: Symptoms or functional impairment between "mild" and "severe."

3-Severe, without Psychotic Features: Several symptoms in excess of those required to make the diagnosis, **and** symptoms markedly interfere with occupational functioning or with usual social activities or relationships with others.

4-With Psychotic Features: Delusions or hallucinations. If possible, **specify** whether the psychotic features are mood-congruent or mood-incongruent.

Mood-congruent psychotic features: Delusions or hallucinations whose content is entirely consistent with the typical depressive themes of personal inadequacy, guilt, disease, death, nihilism, or deserved punishment.

Mood-incongruent psychotic features: Delusions or hallucinations whose content does not involve typical depressive themes of personal inadequacy, guilt, disease, death, nihilism, or deserved punishment.

Included here are such symptoms as persecutory delusions (not directly related to depressive themes), thought insertion, thought broadcasting, and delusions of control.

5-In Partial Remission: Intermediate between "In Full Remission" and "Mild," **and** no previous Dysthymia. (If Major Depressive Episode was superimposed on Dysthymia, the diagnosis of Dysthymia alone is given once the full criteria for a Major Depressive Episode are no longer met.)

6-In Full Remission: During the past six months no significant signs or symptoms of the disturbance.

0-Unspecified.

Specify chronic if current episode has lasted two consecutive years without a period of two months or longer during which there were no significant depressive symptoms.

Specify if current episode is **Melancholic Type.**

Diagnostic criteria for Melancholic Type

The presence of at least five of the following:

(1) loss of interest or pleasure in all, or almost all, activities
(2) lack of reactivity to usually pleasurable stimuli (does not feel much better, even temporarily, when something good happens)
(3) depression regularly worse in the morning
(4) early morning awakening (at least two hours before usual time of awakening)
(5) psychomotor retardation or agitation (not merely subjective complaints)
(6) significant anorexia or weight loss (e.g., more than 5% of body weight in a month)
(7) no significant personality disturbance before first Major Depressive Episode
(8) one or more previous Major Depressive Episodes followed by complete, or nearly complete, recovery
(9) previous good response to specific and adequate somatic antidepressant therapy, e.g., tricyclics, ECT, MAOI, lithium

Diagnostic criteria for seasonal pattern

A. There has been a regular temporal relationship between the onset of an episode of Bipolar Disorder (including Bipolar Disorder NOS) or Recurrent Major Depression (including Depressive Disorder NOS) and a particular 60-day period of the year (e.g., regular appearance of depression between the beginning of October and the end of November).

Note: Do not include cases in which there is an obvious effect of seasonally related psychosocial stressors, e.g., regularly being unemployed every winter.

B. Full remissions (or a change from depression to mania or hypomania) also occurred within a particular 60-day period of the year (e.g., depression disappears from mid-February to mid-April).

C. There have been at least three episodes of mood disturbance in three separate years that demonstrated the temporal seasonal relationship defined in A and B; at least two of the years were consecutive.

D. Seasonal episodes of mood disturbance, as described above, outnumbered any nonseasonal episodes of such disturbance that may have occurred by more than three to one.

Diagnostic criteria for Dysthymia

A. Depressed mood (or can be irritable mood in children and adolescents) for most of the day, more days than not, as indicated either by subjective account or observation by others, for at least two years (one year for children and adolescents).

B. Presence, while depressed, of at least two of the following:

   (1) poor appetite or overeating
   (2) insomnia or hypersomnia
   (3) low energy or fatigue
   (4) low self-esteem
   (5) poor concentration or difficulty making decisions
   (6) feelings of hopelessness

C. During a two-year period (one-year for children and adolescents) of the disturbance, never without the symptoms in A for more than two months at a time.

D. No evidence of an unequivocal Major Depressive Episode during the first two years (one year for children and adolescents) of the disturbance.

Note: There may have been a previous Major Depressive Episode, provided there was a full remission (no significant signs or symptoms for six months) before development of the Dysthymia. In addition, after these two years (one year in children or adolescents) of Dysthymia, there may be superimposed episodes of Major Depression, in which case both diagnoses are given.

E. Has never had a Manic Episode or an unequivocal Hypomanic Episode.

F. Not superimposed on a chronic psychotic disorder, such as Schizophrenia or Delusional Disorder.

G. It cannot be established that an organic factor initiated and maintained the disturbance, e.g., prolonged administration of an antihypertensive medication.

Specify primary or **secondary type:**

Primary type: The mood disturbance is not related to a preexisting, chronic, nonmood, Axis I or Axis III disorder, e.g., Anorexia Nervosa, Somatization Disorder, a Psychoactive Substance Dependence Disorder, an Anxiety Disorder, or rheumatoid arthritis.

Secondary type: the mood disturbance is apparently related to a preexisting, chronic, nonmood Axis I or Axis III disorder.

Specify early onset or **late onset:**

Early onset: onset of the disturbance before age 21.

Late onset: onset of the disturbance at age 21 or later.

Diagnostic criteria for Manic Episode

Note: A "Manic Syndrome" is defined as including criteria A, B, and C below. A "Hypomanic Syndrome" is defined as including criteria A and B, but not C, i.e., no marked impairment.

A. A distinct period of abnormally and persistently elevated, expansive, or irritable mood.

B. During the period of mood disturbance, at least three of the following symptoms have persisted (four if the mood is only irritable) and have been present to a significant degree:

(1) inflated self-esteem or grandiosity
(2) decreased need for sleep, e.g., feels rested after only three hours of sleep

(3) more talkative than usual or pressure to keep talking

(4) flight of ideas or subjective experience that thoughts are racing

(5) distractability, i.e., attention too easily drawn to unimportant or irrelevant external stimuli

(6) increase in goal-directed activity (either socially, at work or school, or sexually) or psychomotor agitation

(7) excessive involvement in pleasurable activities which have a high potential for painful consequences, e.g., the person engages in unrestrained buying sprees, sexual indiscretions, or foolish business investments

C. Mood disturbance sufficiently severe to cause marked impairment in occupational functioning or in usual social activities or relationships with others, or to necessitate hospitalization to prevent harm to self or others.

D. At no time during the disturbance have there been delusions or hallucinations for as long as two weeks in the absence of prominent mood symptoms (i.e., before the mood symptoms developed or after they have remitted).

E. Not superimposed on Schizophrenia, Schizophreniform Disorder, Delusional Disorder, or Psychotic Disorder NOS.

F. It cannot be established that an organic factor initiated and maintained the disturbance. Note: Somatic antidepressant treatment (e.g., drugs, ECT) that apparently precipitates a mood disturbance should not be considered an etiologic organic factor.

Manic Episode codes: Criteria for severity of current state of Bipolar Disorder, Manic or Mixed:

1-Mild: Meets minimum symptom criteria for a Manic Episode (or almost meets symptom criteria if there has been a previous Manic Episode).

2-Moderate: Extreme increase in activity or impairment in judgment.

3-Severe, without Psychotic Features: Almost continual supervision required in order to prevent physical harm to self or others.

4-With Psychotic Features: Delusions, hallucinations, or catatonic symptoms. If possible, specify whether the psychotic features are mood-congruent or mood-incongruent.

Mood-congruent psychotic features: Delusions or hallucinations whose content is entirely consistent with the typical manic themes of inflated worth, power, knowledge, identity, or special relationship to a deity or famous person.

Mood-incongruent psychotic features: Either (a) or (b):

(a) Delusions or hallucinations whose content does not involve the typical manic themes of inflated worth, power, knowledge, identity, or special relationship to a deity or famous person. Included are such symptoms as persecutory delusions (not directly related to grandiose ideas or themes), thought insertion, and delusions of being controlled.

(b) Catatonic symptoms, e.g., stupor, mutism, negativism, posturing.

5-In Partial Remission: Full criteria were previously, but are not currently, met; some signs or symptoms of the disturbance have persisted.

6-In Full Remission: Full criteria were previously met, but there have been no significant signs or symptoms of the disturbance for at least six months.

0-Unspecified.

Diagnostic criteria for Bipolar Disorders

Bipolar Disorder, Mixed

Use the Manic Episode codes to describe current state.

A. Current (or most recent) episode involves the full symptomatic picture of both Manic and Major Depressive Episodes (except for the duration requirement of two weeks for depressive symptoms), intermixed or rapidly alternating every few days.

B. Prominent depressive symptoms lasting at least a full day.

Specify if **seasonal pattern.**

Bipolar Disorder, Manic

Use the Manic Episode codes to describe current state.

Currently (or most recently) in a Manic Episode. (If there has been a previous Manic Episode, the current episode need not meet the full criteria for a Manic Episode.)

Specify if **seasonal pattern.**

Bipolar Disorder, Depressed

Use the Major Depressive Episode codes to describe current state.

A. Has had one or more Manic Episodes.

B. Currently (or most recently) in a Major Depressive Episode. (If there has been a previous Major Depressive Episode, the current episode need not meet the full criteria for a Major Depressive Episode.)

Specify if **seasonal pattern.**

Diagnostic criteria for Cyclothymia

A. For at least two years (one year for children and adolescents), presence of numerous Hypomanic Episodes (all of the criteria for a Manic Episode, except criterion C that indicates marked impairment) and numerous periods with depressed mood or loss of interest or pleasure that did not meet criterion A of Major Depressive Episode.

B. During a two-year period (one-year in children and adolescents) of the disturbance, never without hypomanic or depressive symptoms for more than two months at a time.

C. No clear evidence of a Major Depressive Episode or Manic Episode during the first two years of the disturbance (or one year in children and adolescents).

Note: After this minimum period of Cyclothymia, there may be superimposed Manic or Major Depressive Episodes, in which case the additional diagnosis of Bipolar Disorder or Bipolar Disorder NOS should be given.

D. Not superimposed on a chronic psychotic disorder, such as Schizophrenia or Delusional Disorder.

E. It cannot be established that an organic factor initiated and maintained the disturbance, e.g., repeated intoxication from drugs or alcohol.

Diagnostic criteria for Delirium

A. Reduced ability to maintain attention to external stimuli (e.g., questions must be repeated because attention wanders) and to appropriately shift attention to new external stimuli (e.g., perseverates answer to a previous question).

B. Disorganized thinking, as indicated by rambling, irrelevant, or incoherent speech.

C. At least two of the following:

(1) reduced level of consciousness, e.g., difficulty keeping awake during examination

(2) perceptual disturbances: misinterpretations, illusions, or hallucinations

(3) disturbance of sleep-wake cycle with insomnia or daytime sleepiness

(4) increased or decreased psychomotor activity

(5) disorientation to time, place, or person

(6) memory impairment, e.g., inability to learn new material, such as the names of several unrelated objects after five minutes, or to remember past events, such as history of current episode of illness

D. Clinical features develop over a short period of time (usually hours to days) and tend to fluctuate over the course of a day.

E. Either (1) or (2):

(1) evidence from the history, physical examination, or laboratory tests of a specific organic factor (or factors) judged to be etiologically related to the disturbance

(2) in the absence of such evidence, an etiologic organic factor can be presumed if the disturbance cannot be accounted for by any nonorganic mental disorder, e.g., Manic Episode accounting for agitation and sleep disturbance

Diagnostic criteria for Dementia

A. Demonstrable evidence of impairment in short- and long-term memory. Impairment in short-term memory (inability to learn new information) may be indicated by inability to remember three objects after five minutes. Long-term memory impairment (inability to remember information that was known in the past) may be indicated by inability to remember past personal information (e.g., what happened yesterday, birthplace, occupation) or facts of common knowledge (e.g., past Presidents, well-known dates.)

B. At least one of the following:

(1) impairment in abstract thinking, as indicated by inability to find similarities and differences between related words, difficulty in defining words and concepts, and other similar tasks

(2) impaired judgment, as indicated by inability to make reasonable plans to deal with interpersonal, family, and job-related problems and issues

(3) other disturbances of higher cortical function, such as aphasia (disorder of language), apraxia (inability to carry out motor activities despite intact comprehension and motor function),

agnosia (failure to recognize or identify objects despite intact sensory function), and "constructional difficulty" (e.g., inability to copy three-dimensional figures, assemble blocks, or arrange sticks in specific designs)

(4) personality change, i.e., alteration or accentuation of premorbid traits

C. The disturbance in A and B significantly interferes with work or usual social activities or relationships with others.

D. Not occurring exclusively during the course of Delirium.

E. Either (1) or (2):

(1) there is evidence from the history, physical examination, or laboratory tests of a specific organic factor (or factors) judged to be etiologically related to the disturbance

(2) in the absence of such evidence, an etiologic organic factor can be presumed if the disturbance cannot be accounted for by any nonorganic mental disorder, e.g., Major Depression accounting for cognitive impairment

Criteria for severity of Dementia:

Mild: Although work or social activities are significantly impaired, the capacity for independent living remains, with adequate personal hygiene and relatively intact judgment.

Moderate: Independent living is hazardous, and some degree of supervision is necessary.

Severe: Activities of daily living are so impaired that continual supervision is required, e.g., unable to maintain minimal personal hygiene; largely incoherent or mute.

Diagnostic criteria for Primary Degenerative Dementia of the Alzheimer Type

A. Dementia.

B. Insidious onset with a generally progressive deteriorating course.

C. Exclusion of all other specific causes of Dementia by history, physical examination, and laboratory tests.

Diagnostic criteria for Multi-infarct Dementia

A. Dementia.

B. Stepwise deteriorating course with "patchy" distribution of deficits (i.e., affecting some functions, but not others) early in the course.

C. Focal neuralgic signs and symptoms (e.g., exaggeration of deep tendon reflexes, extensor plantar response, pseudobulbar palsy, gait abnormalities, weakness of an extremity, etc.).

D. Evidence from history, physical examination, or laboratory tests of significant cerebrovascular disease (recorded on Axis III) that is judged to be etiologically related to the disturbance.

Diagnostic criteria for Psychoactive Substance Dependence

A. At least three of the following:

(1) substance often taken in larger amounts or over a longer period than the person intended

(2) persistent desire or one or more unsuccessful efforts to cut down or control substance use

(3) a great deal of time spent in activities necessary to get the substance (e.g., theft), taking the substance (e.g., chain smoking), or recovering from its effects

(4) frequent intoxication or withdrawal symptoms when expected to fulfill major role obligations at work, school, or home (e.g., does not go to work because hung over, goes to school or work "high," intoxicated while taking care of his or her children), or when substance use is physically hazardous (e.g., drives when intoxicated)

(5) important social, occupational, or recreational activities given up or reduced because of substance use

(6) continued substance use despite knowledge of having a persistent or recurrent social, psychological, or physical problem that is caused or exacerbated by the use of the substance (e.g., keeps using heroin despite family arguments about it, cocaine-induced depression, or having an ulcer made worse by drinking)

(7) marked tolerance: need for markedly increased amounts of the substance (i.e., at least 50% increase) in order to achieve intoxication or desired effect, or markedly diminished effect with continued use of the same amount

Note: The following items may not apply to cannabis, hallucinogens, or phencyclidine (PCP):

(8) characteristic withdrawal symptoms (see specific withdrawal syndromes under Psychoactive Substance-induced Organic Mental Disorders)

(9) substance often taken to relieve or avoid withdrawal symptoms

B. Some symptoms of the disturbance have persisted for at least one month, or have occurred repeatedly over a longer period of time.

Criteria for severity of Psychoactive Substance Dependence:

Mild: Few, if any, symptoms in excess of those required to make the diagnosis, and the symptoms result in no more than mild impairment in occupational functioning or in usual social activities or relationships with others.

Moderate: Symptoms or functional impairment between "mild" and "severe."

Severe: Many symptoms in excess of those required to make the diagnosis, and the symptoms markedly interfere with occupational functioning or with usual social activities or relationships with others. (Because of the availability of cigarettes and other nicotine-containing substances and the absence of a clinically significant nicotine intoxication syndrome, impairment in occupational or social functioning is not necessary for a rating of severe Nicotine Dependence.)

In Partial Remission: During the past six months, some use of the substance and some symptoms of dependence.

In Full Remission: During the past six months, either no use of the substance, or use of the substance and no symptoms of dependence.

Diagnostic criteria for Psychoactive Substance Abuse

A. A maladaptive pattern of psychoactive substance use indicated by at least one of the following:

(1) continued use despite the knowledge of having a persistent or recurrent social, occupational, psychological, or physical problem that is caused or exacerbated by use of the psychoactive substance

(2) recurrent use in situations in which use is physically hazardous (e.g., driving while intoxicated)

B. Some symptoms of the disturbance have persisted for at least one month, or have occurred repeatedly over a longer period of time.

C. Never met the criteria for Psychoactive Substance Dependence for this substance.

Diagnostic criteria for Schizophrenia

A. Presence of characteristic psychotic symptoms in the active phase: either (1), (2), or (3) for at least one week (unless the symptoms are successfully treated):

(1) two of the following:

(a) delusions
(b) prominent hallucinations (throughout the day for several days or several times a week for several weeks, each hallucinatory experience not being limited to a few brief moments)
(c) incoherence or marked loosening of associations
(d) catatonic behavior
(e) flat or grossly inappropriate affect

(2) bizarre delusions (i.e., involving a phenomenon that the person's culture would regard as totally implausible, e.g., thought broadcasting, being controlled by a dead person)

(3) prominent hallucinations [as defined in (1)(b) above] of a voice with content having no apparent relation to depression or elation, or a voice keeping up a running commentary on the person's behavior or thoughts, or two or more voices conversing with each other

B. During the course of the disturbance, functioning in such areas as work, social relations, and self-care is markedly below the highest level achieved before onset of the disturbance (or, when the onset is in childhood or adolescence, failure to achieve expected level of social development).

C. Schizoaffective Disorder and Mood Disorder with Psychotic Features have been ruled out, i.e., if a Major Depressive or Manic Syndrome has ever been present during an active phase of the disturbance, the total duration of all episodes of a mood syndrome has been brief relative to the total duration of the active and residual phases of the disturbance.

D. Continuous signs of the disturbance for at least six months. The six-month period must include an active phase (of at least one week, or less if symptoms have been successfully treated) during which there were psychotic symptoms characteristic of Schizophrenia (symptoms in A), with or without a prodromal or residual phase, as defined below.

Prodromal phase: A clear deterioration in functioning before the active phase of the disturbance that is not due to a disturbance in mood or to a Psychoactive Substance Use Disorder and that involves at least two of the symptoms listed below.

Residual phase: Following the active phase of the disturbance, persistence of at least two of the symptoms noted below, these not being due to a disturbance in mood or to a Psychoactive Substance Use Disorder.

Prodromal or Residual Symptoms:

(1) marked social isolation or withdrawal
(2) marked impairment in role functioning as wage-earner, student, or homemaker
(3) markedly peculiar behavior (e.g., collecting garbage, talking to self in public, hoarding food)
(4) marked impairment in personal hygiene and grooming
(5) blunted or inappropriate affect
(6) digressive, vague, overelaborate, or circumstantial speech, or poverty of speech, or poverty of content of speech
(7) odd beliefs or magical thinking, influencing behavior and inconsistent with cultural norms, e.g., superstitiousness, belief in clairvoyance, telepathy, "sixth sense," "others can feel my feelings," overvalued ideas, ideas of reference
(8) unusual perceptual experiences, e.g., recurrent illusions, sensing the presence of a force or person not actually present
(9) marked lack of initiative, interests, or energy

Examples: Six months of prodromal symptoms with one week of symptoms from A; no prodromal symptoms with six months of symptoms from A; no prodromal symptoms with one week of symptoms from A and six months of residual symptoms.

E. It cannot be established that an organic factor initiated and maintained the disturbance.

F. If there is a history of Autistic Disorder, the additional diagnosis of Schizophrenia is made only if prominent delusions or hallucinations are also present.

Classification of course:

1-Subchronic. The time from the beginning of the disturbance, when the person first began to show signs of the disturbance (including prodromal, active, and residual phases) more or less continuously, is less than two years, but at least six months.

2-Chronic. Same as above, but more than two years.

3-Subchronic with Acute Exacerbation. Reemergence of prominent psychotic symptoms in a person with a subchronic course who has been in the residual phase of the disturbance.

4-Chronic with Acute Exacerbation. Reemergence of prominent psychotic symptoms in a person with a chronic course who has been in the residual phase of the disturbance.

5-In Remission. When a person with a history of Schizophrenia is free of all signs of the disturbance (whether or not on medication), "In Remission" should be coded. Differentiating Schizophrenia in Remission from No Mental Disorder requires consideration of overall level of functioning, length of time since the last episode of disturbance, total duration of the disturbance, and whether prophylactic treatment is being given.

0-Unspecified.

Diagnostic criteria for Delusional Disorder

A. Nonbizarre delusion(s) (i.e., involving situations that occur in real life, such as being followed, poisoned, infected, loved at a distance, having a disease, being deceived by one's spouse or lover) of at least one month's duration.

B. Auditory or visual hallucinations, if present, are not prominent [as defined in Schizophrenia, A(1)(b)].

C. Apart from the delusion(s) or its ramifications, behavior is not obviously odd or bizarre.

D. If a Major Depressive or Manic Syndrome has been present during the delusional disturbance, the total duration of all episodes of the mood syndrome has been brief relative to the total duration of the delusional disturbance.

E. Has never met criterion A for schizophrenia, and it cannot be established that an organic factor initiated and maintained the disturbance.

Specify type: The following types are based on the predominant delusional theme. If no single delusional theme predominates, specify as **Unspecified Type.**

Erotomanic Type
Delusional Disorder in which the predominant theme of the delusion(s) is that a person, usually of higher status, is in love with the subject.

Grandiose Type
Delusional Disorder in which the predominant theme of the delusion(s) is one of inflated worth, power, knowledge, identity, or special relationship to a deity or famous person.

Jealous Type
Delusional Disorder in which the predominant theme of the delusion(s) is that one's sexual partner is unfaithful.

Persecutory Type
Delusional Disorder in which the predominant theme of the delusion(s) is that one (or someone to whom one is close) is being malevolently treated in some way. People with this type of Delusional Disorder may repeatedly take their complaints of being mistreated to legal authorities.

Somatic Type
Delusional Disorder in which the predominant theme of the delusion(s) is that the person has some physical defect, disorder, or disease.

Unspecified Type
Delusional Disorder that does not fit any of the previous categories, e.g., persecutory and grandiose themes without a predominance of either; delusions of reference without malevolent content.

Diagnostic criteria for Panic Disorder

A. At some time during the disturbance, one or more panic attacks (discrete periods of intense fear or discomfort) have occurred that were (1) unexpected, i.e., did not occur immediately before or on exposure to a situation that almost always caused anxiety, and (2) not triggered by situations in which the person was the focus of others' attention.

B. Either four attacks, as defined in criterion A, have occurred within a four-week period, or one or more attacks have been followed by a period of at least a month of persistent fear of having another attack.

C. At least four of the following symptoms developed during at least one of the attacks:

(1) shortness of breath (dyspnea) or smothering sensations
(2) dizziness, unsteady feelings, or faintness
(3) palpitations or accelerated heart rate (tachycardia)
(4) trembling or shaking
(5) sweating
(6) choking
(7) nausea or abdominal distress
(8) depersonalization or derealization
(9) numbness or tingling sensations (paresthesias)
(10) flushes (hot flashes) or chills
(11) chest pain or discomfort
(12) fear of dying
(13) fear of going crazy or of doing something uncontrolled

Note: Attacks involving four or more symptoms are panic attacks; attacks involving fewer than four symptoms are limited symptom attacks (see Agoraphobia without History of Panic Disorder).

D. During at least some of the attacks, at least four of the C symptoms developed suddenly and increased in intensity within ten minutes of the beginning of the first C symptom noticed in the attack.

E. It cannot be established that an organic factor initiated and maintained the disturbance, e.g., Amphetamine or Caffeine Intoxication, hyperthyroidism.

Note: Mitral valve prolapse may be an associated condition, but does not preclude a diagnosis of Panic Disorder.

Diagnostic criteria for Panic Disorder with Agoraphobia

A. Meets the criteria for Panic Disorder.

B. Agoraphobia: Fear of being in places or situations from which escape might be difficult (or embarrassing) or in which help might not be available in the event of a panic attack. (Include cases in which persistent avoidance behavior originated during an active phase of Panic Disorder, even if the person does not attribute the avoidance behavior to fear of having a panic attack.) As a result of this fear, the person either restricts travel or needs a companion when away from home, or else endures agoraphobic situations despite intense anxiety. Common agoraphobic situations include being outside the home alone, being in a crowd or standing in line, being on a bridge, and traveling in a bus, train, or car.

Specify current severity of agoraphobic avoidance:

Mild: Some avoidance (or endurance with distress), but relatively normal lifestyle, e.g., travels unaccompanied when necessary, such as to work or to shop; otherwise avoids traveling alone.

Moderate: Avoidance results in constricted lifestyle, e.g., the person is able to leave the house alone, but not to go more than a few miles unaccompanied.

Severe: Avoidance results in being nearly or completely housebound or unable to leave the house unaccompanied.

In Partial Remission: No current agoraphobic avoidance, but some agoraphobic avoidance during the past six months.

In Full Remission: No current agoraphobic avoidance and none during the past six months.

Specify current severity of panic attacks:

Mild: During the past month, either all attacks have been limited symptom attacks (i.e., fewer than four symptoms), or there has been no more than one panic attack.

Moderate: During the past month attacks have been intermediate between "mild" and "severe."

Severe: During the past month, there have been at least eight panic attacks.

In Partial Remission: The condition has been intermediate between "In Full Remission" and "Mild."

In Full Remission: During the past six months, there have been no panic or limited symptom attacks.

Diagnostic criteria for Panic Disorder without Agoraphobia

A. Meets the criteria for Panic Disorder.

B. Absence of Agoraphobia, as defined above.

Specify current severity of panic attacks, as defined above.

Diagnostic criteria for Social Phobia

A. A persistent fear of one or more situations (the social phobic situations) in which the person is exposed to possible scrutiny by others and fears that he or she may do something or act in a way that will be humiliating or embarrassing. Examples include: being unable to continue talking while speaking in public, choking on food when eating in front of others, being unable to urinate in a public lavatory, hand-trembling when writing in the presence of others, and saying foolish things or not being able to answer questions in social situations.

B. If an Axis III or another Axis I disorder is present, the fear in A is unrelated to it, e.g., the fear is not of having a panic attack (Panic Disorder), stuttering (Stuttering), trembling (Parkinson's disease), or exhibiting abnormal eating behaviors (Anorexia Nervosa or Bulimia Nervosa).

C. During some phase of the disturbance, exposure to the specific phobic stimulus (or stimuli) almost invariably provokes an immediate anxiety response.

D. The phobic situations(s) is avoided, or is endured with intense anxiety.

E. The avoidant behavior interferes with occupational functioning or with usual social activities or relationships with others, or there is marked distress about having the fear.

F. The person recognizes that his or her fear is excessive or unreasonable.

G. If the person is under 18, the disturbance does not meet the criteria for Avoidant Disorder of Childhood or Adolescence.

Specify generalized type if the phobic situation includes most social situations, and also consider the additional diagnosis of Avoidant Personality Disorder.

Diagnostic criteria for Simple Phobia

A. A persistent fear of a circumscribed stimulus (object or situation) other than fear of having a panic attack (as in Panic Disorder) or of humiliation or embarrassment in certain social situations (as in Social Phobia).

   Note: Do not include fears that are part of Panic Disorder with Agoraphobia or Agoraphobia without History of Panic Disorder.

B. During some phase of the disturbance, exposure to the specific phobic stimulus (or stimuli) almost invariably provokes an immediate anxiety response.

C. The object or situation is avoided, or endured with intense anxiety.

D. The fear or the avoidant behavior significantly interferes with the person's normal routine or with usual social activities or relationships with others, or there is marked distress about having the fear.

E. The person recognizes that his or her fear is excessive or unreasonable.

F. The phobic stimulus is unrelated to the content of the obsessions of Obsessive Compulsive Disorder or the trauma of Post-traumatic Stress Disorder.

Diagnostic criteria for Obsessive Compulsive Disorder

A. Either obsessions or compulsions:

   Obsessions: (1), (2), (3), and (4):

   (1) recurrent and persistent ideas, thoughts, impulses, or images that are experienced, at least initially, as intrusive and senseless, e.g., a parent's having repeated impulses to kill a loved child, a religious person's having recurrent blasphemous thoughts
   (2) the person attempts to ignore or suppress such thoughts or impulses or to neutralize them with some other thought or action
   (3) the person recognizes that the obsessions are the product of his or her own mind, not imposed from without (as in thought insertion)
   (4) if another Axis I disorder is present, the content of the obsession is unrelated to it, e.g., the ideas, thoughts, impulses, or images are

not about food in the presence of an Eating Disorder, about drugs in the presence of a Psychoactive Substance Use Disorder, or guilty thoughts in the presence of a Major Depression.

Compulsions: (1), (2), and (3):

(1) repetitive, purposeful, and intentional behaviors that are performed in response to an obsession, or according to certain rules or in a stereotyped fashion

(2) the behavior is designed to neutralize or to prevent discomfort or some dreaded event or situation; however, either the activity is not connected in a realistic way with what it is designed to neutralize or prevent, or it is clearly excessive

(3) the person recognizes that his or her behavior is excessive or unreasonable (this may not be true for young children; it may no longer be true for people whose obsessions have evolved into overvalued ideas)

B. The obsessions or compulsions cause marked distress, are time-consuming (take more than an hour a day), or significantly interfere with the person's normal routine, occupational functioning, or usual social activities or relationships with others.

Diagnostic criteria for Generalized Anxiety Disorder

A. Unrealistic or excessive anxiety and worry (apprehensive expectation) about two or more life circumstances, e.g., worry about possible misfortune to one's child (who is in no danger) and worry about finances (for no good reason), for a period of six months or longer, during which the person has been bothered more days than not by these concerns. In children and adolescents, this may take the form of anxiety and worry about academic, athletic, and social performance.

B. If another Axis I disorder is present, the focus of the anxiety and worry in A is unrelated to it, e.g., the anxiety or worry is not about having a panic attack (as in Panic Disorder), being embarrassed in public (as in Social Phobia), being contaminated (as in Obsessive Compulsive Disorder), or gaining weight (as in Anorexia Nervosa).

C. The disturbance does not occur only during the course of a Mood Disorder or a psychotic disorder.

D. At least 6 of the following 18 symptoms are often present when anxious (do not include symptoms present only during panic attacks):

Motor tension

(1) trembling, twitching, or feeling shaky
(2) muscle tension, aches, or soreness

(3) restlessness
(4) easy fatigability

Autonomic hyperactivity

(5) shortness of breath or smothering sensations
(6) palpitations or accelerated heart rate (tachycardia)
(7) sweating, or cold clammy hands
(8) dry mouth
(9) dizziness or lightheadedness
(10) nausea, diarrhea, or other abdominal distress
(11) flushes (hot flashes) or chills
(12) frequent urination
(13) trouble swallowing or "lump in throat"

Vigilance and scanning

(14) feeling keyed up or on edge
(15) exaggerated startle response
(16) difficulty concentrating or "mind going blank" because of anxiety
(17) trouble falling or staying asleep
(18) irritability

E. It cannot be established that an organic factor initiated and maintained the disturbance, e.g., hyperthyroidism, Caffeine Intoxication.

Index

AA. *See* Alchoholics Anonymous
AAAs. *See* Area Agencies on Aging
AAGP. *See* American Association for
    Geriatric Psychiatry
AARP. *See* American Association of Retired
    Persons
AARP Pharmacy Service, 177
ACTH. *See* Adrenocorticotropic hormone
Acute dystonic reaction, 121
ADRCs. *See* Alzheimer's Disease Research
    Centers
Adrenocorticotropic hormone (ACTH), 94
Adult Development and Aging, 230
Advocacy groups, 164, 176, 177, 184, 185
    mental health, 182, 187
Age Page: Aging and Alcohol Abuse, 240
*Age Page: Safe Use of Medicines in Older
    People,* 240
Age Page: Safe Use of Tranquilizers, 240
Age Page: Senility: Myth or Madness?, 240
Age Page: When You Need a Nursing Home,
    240
Age Page: Who's Who in Health Care, 240
Age Pages, 239–240
Aging, 221, 226, 227, 233–235, 242
    of brain, 70–71
    and depression, 222, 233
    general reading on, 228–231
*Aging and Mental Disorders: Psychological
    Approaches to Assessment and
    Treatment,* 228
Aging and Mental Health, 233
*Aging and Mental Health: Positive
    Psychosocial and Biomedical
    Approaches,* 223
Agnosia, 75
Agoraphobia, 107, 126–127, 129
AGS. *See* American Geriatrics Society
Akathisia, 121

Akinesia, 121
Alcohol, 79, 84, 108
    abuse of, 244–245
    body's use of, 140–141
    use of, 135–138
    See also Alchoholism
*Alcohol, Drugs, and Seniors: Tarnished
    Dreams* (video/film), 244–245
Alcohol rehabilitation programs, 109
Alcoholics Anonymous (AA), 142, 175
Alcoholism, 75, 84, 109
    causes of, 138–140
    See also Alcohol; Substance use disorders
Allergies, 29
Aluminum, 82
Alzheimer, Alois, 71
*The Alzheimer Caregiver: Strategies for
    Support,* 227
Alzheimer's Association, 72, 101, 164,
    175–176
    pamphlets, 236–237
Alzheimer's disease, 68, 69, 75, 76, 87, 91,
    101, 102, 241, 243, 247–248
    causes of, 80–81
    frequency, 77, 78
    impact on family of, 91–92, 228,
    234–235, 248–249
    pamphlets on, 236–237
    patient care, 224, 233–234, 245–246
    research, 186–187
    treatment of, 94–95
Alzheimer's Disease: A Guide for Families, 234
Alzheimer's Disease: An Overview, 236
Alzheimer's Disease: Services You May Need,
    236
*Alzheimer's Disease Research Center
    Program List,* 241
Alzheimer's Disease Research Centers
    (ADRCs), 186–187, 188–190, 241

American Association for Geriatric
   Psychiatry (AAGP), 176, 225
American Association of Retired Persons
   (AARP), 177
American Board of Psychiatry and
   Neurology, 166
American Geriatrics Society (AGS), 177–178
American Psychiatric Association (APA),
   178–179
   local societies, 190–195
   pamphlets, 237–239
American Psychiatric Press, 179
American Psychological Association (APA)
   state associations, 195–198
American Society on Aging (ASA), 179–180
Amobarbital, 133
Amoxapine, 42
Amphetamines, 94
Amytal, 133
Anafranil, 133
Anemia, 79
Aneurysms, 83
Antabuse, 142
Anti-anxiety drugs, 42
Anticholinergic effects, 39, 121
Antidepressants, 36–37
   for anxiety, 132–133
   atypical, 41–42
   lithium as, 42
   monoamine oxidase inhibitors as, 40–41
   for pseudodementia, 93
   tricyclic, 37–40, 95
Antihistamines, 133
Anxiety, 125
Anxiety and Its Treatment: Help Is Available,
   232
Anxiety disorders, 237
   definitions of, 125–129
   evaluation for, 130–131
   frequency of, 129–130
   treatment of, 107–108, 131–134, 232
   types of, 106–107
Anxiolytics, 142
   dependence on, 108, 109, 135, 141
APA. *See* American Psychiatric Association;
   American Psychological Association
Aphasia, 75
Appetite, as symptom of major depression, 9
Apraxia, 75
Area Agencies on Aging, 153
   service coordination, 159–160, 164

ASA. *See* American Society on Aging
Ascendin, 42
Aspirin, 93
Assisting the Person with Alzheimer's, 236
Ativan, 131
Autism, 113

Barbiturates, 133
Beale, Caroline T., 231
Beck, Aaron, 23, 50
Behavior
   and anxiety, 130
   and depression, 21–24
   and emotions, 50–51
Behavior therapy, 50–51
Benadryl, 122, 133
Benzodiazepines, 95
   for anxiety disorders, 131–132
Benztropine mesylate, 122
Bereavement, and depression, 10, 12, 18–19
Bernheim, Kayla F., 231
Beta-blockers, 132
Billig, Nathan, 233
Binstock, Robert H., 221
Bipolar disorder, 4–6, 60, 119, 238, 239,
   241, 246–247
   definition of, 57–58
   lithium treatment for, 61–65
   treatment effectiveness, 64–65
Bipolar Disorder: Manic-Depressive Illness,
   241
Birren, James E., 222
Blazer, Dan, 140, 222
Blood pressure, 121
   and beta-blockers, 132
   and tricyclic antidepressants, 38–39
Board and care facilities, 150
Brain
   abnormal changes in, 71–72
   aging of, 70–71
   chemistry of, 118, 120–121
   injuries to, 83
Brain chemistry
   and depression, 15–17
Brain disorders
   as cause of delirium, 79
   as cause of dementia, 84
Brandts, Wendy, 235
Brannon, Diane, 228
Breslau, Lawrence D., 222
Bupropion, 42

Busse, Ewald W., 222
Butler, Robert N., 29–30, 49, 223, 228, 233

Cancer, pancreatic, 27
Carbamazepine, 63
Cardiac changes, with tricyclic
    antidepressants, 38
Cardiac disease, and electroconvulsive
    therapy, 44
*Care of Alzheimer's Patients: A Manual for
    Nursing Home Staff,* 224
Caregivers, 91, 164, 234, 247, 249–250
    of dementia patients, 98–101, 227,
        233–234, 236, 245–246
Caregiving at Home, 236
*Caring: Families Coping with Alzheimer's
    Disease* (video), 245
*The Caring Family: Living with Chronic
    Mental Illness,* 231
*Caring . . . Sharing: The Alzheimer's
    Caregiver* (video), 245–246
Carstensen, Laura L., 223
Case managers, 167
*The Case of John R.: Depression among
    Older Persons* (video), 246
Case workers, 167
Catatonic behavior, in schizophrenia, 112
Central nervous system anticholinergic
    toxicity, 121
Cerebrovascular disease, 76–77, 79
Chaisson-Stewart, Maureen G., 223
Chlorpromazine, 120
Choline acetyltransferase, 80
*Choosing a Nursing Home: A Guidebook for
    Families,* 235
Clearinghouses, 188
    self-help, 215–218
Clinical Geriatric Psychopharmacology, 227
Clinics. *See* Community mental health
    centers; Geriatric Research, Education,
    and Clinical Centers
Clomipramine, 133
CMHCs. *See* Community mental health
    centers
Cogentin, 122
Cognition
    assessing, 87–88
    changes in, 32–33
    and depression, 23–24, 32–33, 88–89
    loss of, 69–71, 102
    problems with, 85–87

Cognitive therapy, for depression, 50–51
Cohen, Donna, 233–234
Cohen, Gene D., 226
Cohn, Margaret D., 228
Cole, Thomas R., 229
Communicating with the Alzheimer Patient, 236
Community agencies, 101, 164
Community Group for the Advancement of
    Psychiatry, 231
Community mental health centers (CMHCs),
    163
    establishment, 148–149
    Medicare, 155
    model programs, 203–205
    organization for, 184–185
    problems with, 149–150
    services, 151–152
Compulsions, 107, 128
Computerized axial transverse tomography
    (CT) scan, 89–90, 118
Concentration problems, as symptom of
    major depression, 9–10
Conceptual disorganization, 110, 119
Constructional difficulties, 75
Consumers, service users as, 165
*A Consumer's Guide to Mental Health
    Services,* 241–242
Control Your Depression, 232
*Coping and Home Safety Tips for Caregivers
    of the Elderly* (video), 246
Costs, of mental health care, 167. *See also*
    Finances
Counseling, 153
    for dementia patients, 96–98
Counselors, mental health, 167
Couples, psychotherapy for, 52–53
Courtice, Katie, 234
Creutzfeldt-Jakob disease, 75, 78, 83
CT scan. *See* Computerized axial transverse
    tomography scan
Cyclandelate, 94
Cyclothymia, 5, 59–60

Dahm, Lynn, 235
Day care, for dementia patients, 164
Death, coping with, 18–19. *See also*
    Bereavement
Delirium, 67
    causes of, 68, 78–79
    characteristics of, 73–74
    from drug toxicity, 141

Delirium *(continued)*
  evaluation for, 86, 87, 89–90
  frequencies, 77–78
  treatment for, 92–93, 96
Delusional disorder, 117, 118
  characteristics of, 105–106
  defined, 113–116
Delusions, 105, 110
  evaluation of, 89, 119
  during manic episodes, 59
  in schizophrenia, 112
  as symptom in major depression, 9–11
  treatment for, 119, 123
Dementia, 67, 101–102, 132, 238, 249
  and brain changes, 71
  care for, 164, 233–234
  causes of, 75–76
  characteristics of, 74–75
  and delirium, 73
  and depression, 95
  drug toxicity, 141
  evaluation for, 86, 89–90, 102–103, 241
  family and treatment, 98–101, 160–161
  frequencies of, 77–78
  irreversible, 79–83
  and medication, 62, 248
  nonprogressive, 83–84
  nursing home care, 224
  primary degenerative, 76
  reversible, 84–85, 92–93
  support services for, 153, 175–176
  supportive counseling for, 96–98
  types of, 68, 76–77
Department of Veterans Affairs (VA)
  clinics, 145, 199–200
  services, 152, 153, 164, 180–181
Departments of mental health/hygiene,
    163
Depression, 6–7, 14, 15, 65, 223, 233,
    237–239, 242, 246
  and age, 12–13, 222
  and alcohol, 139
  and anxiety, 133
  brain chemistry, 15–17
  cognitive and behavioral approach to, 21–24
  cognitive changes, 32–33, 88–89
  contexts of, 29–30
  definition of, 7–8
  and delusional disorders, 114
  and dementia, 84–85, 87, 95

electroconvulsive therapy for, 42–44
environmental stress and, 17–20
frequency of, 13–14
medication as cause, 28–29
medication treatment for, 36–42, 93
psychodynamic approaches to, 20–21
psychotherapy for, 44–54
treatment of, 33–34, 54–57, 231, 232
types of, 3–5, 8–12
See also specific types
Depression: What You Need To Know, 242
*Depression and Aging: Causes, Care, and
    Consequences*, 222
*Depression and Its Treatment: Help for the
    Nation's No. 1 Mental Problem*, 231
*Depression in the Elderly: An
    Interdisciplinary Approach*, 223
*Depressive Disorders: Treatments Bring New
    Hope*, 242
*Depressive Illness: Now You Can Learn How
    To Help*, 239
Depressive Illness Project of the National
    Alliance for the Mentally Ill, 239
Desyrel, 42
Diagnosis, 168
  of dementia or delirium, 89–90, 102–103,
    241
  of mental disorders, 7–8
  of mood disorder, 26–27
Diagnosis-related groups (DRGs), 156
*The Diagnostic and Statistical Manual of
    Mental Disorders*, 7, 8, 13, 26
  on cyclothymia, 59–60
  on delusional disorder, 113–114
  on dementia, 76–77, 86
  on manic episodes, 58–59
  on psychoactive substance dependence,
    136–137
  on schizophrenia, 111–113
  on syndromes and disorders, 72
Diazepam, 131
Diet, and depression medication, 41
*Differential Diagnosis of Dementing
    Diseases: National Institutes of Health
    Consensus Development Conference
    Statement*, 241
Diphenhydramine hydrochloride, 122,
    133
*Directory of Fellowship Programs in
    Geriatric Medicine*, 178

Disorder
  defined, 67, 72
  types of, 105–109
  See also specific types
Disulfiram, 142
Doctors. *See* General practitioners; Private
  practitioners
Dopamine, 83
Double depression, 12
Down's syndrome, and dementia, 80
DRGs. *See* Diagnosis-related groups
Drowsiness, with benzodiazepines, 131
Drugs
  abuse of, 135–136, 138, 140, 244–245
  anti-clotting, 93
  and delirium, 96
  and dementia, 84
  dependence on, 108–109, 138, 140–142
  intoxication from, 79
  metabolization of, 34–36, 120–121
  treatment for dementia, 94–96
  See also Medication; Pharmacological
    treatment; specific drugs
DSM-III-R. *See The Diagnostic and*
  Statistical Manual of Mental Disorders
Dysphoria, 14
Dysthymia, 4, 87
  characteristics of, 11–12

ECT. *See* Electroconvulsive therapy
Edelstein, Barry A., 223
Edinberg, Mark, 223–224, 229
Education, organizations for, 176–177, 187
Eisdorfer, Carl, 233–234
Electroconvulsive therapy (ECT)
  for bipolar disorder, 63
  for depression, 34, 42–44, 57
  for major depression, 3
Emotional distress, 14
Emotions
  and behavior, 50–51
  fluctuation in, 5–6
  in schizophrenia, 112
Endocrine disturbances, as cause of
  dementia, 84
Energy loss, as symptom of major
  depression, 9
Enjoy Old Age: A Program of
  Self-Management, 230–231
Enkephalins, 95

Environment, evaluation of, 90–92
Erikson, Erik H., 229–230
Erikson, Joan M., 229–230
Essentials of Geriatric Psychiatry, 225–226
Evaluation
  of alcoholism, 140–141
  of anxiety disorder, 130–131
  of bipolar disorder, 61
  for cognitive problems, 85–87
  costs of, 167
  for depression, 26–28
  of living environment, 90–92
  of psychotic symptoms, 119
  and rapport, 24–25
  for substance use problems, 140–142
Extrapyramidal effects, from neuroleptics,
  121–122

Fact Sheet: Depression in the Elderly, 242
Family, 231, 232, 247, 249–250
  and dementia patients, 91–92, 98–101,
    228, 233–235, 245, 248–249
  medication monitoring, 142–143
  and mood disorders, 65
  psychotherapy for, 53–54
  services and organizations for, 160–161,
    164, 176, 181, 182
A Family Affair: Helping Families Cope with
  Mental Illness, 231
Family Service America, 152–153, 181
Fatigue, from benzodiazepines, 131
Fellowships, in geriatric psychiatry, 200–203
Fever, as cause of delirium, 79
Films, 244–250
Finances, and care of dementia patients, 99,
  236
Financial Services You May Need, 236
Fluoxetine, 42, 133
Fluphenazine, 120
Fluvoxamine, 133
Four Lives: A Portrait of Manic Depression
  (video/film), 246–247
Freud, Sigmund, 20–21, 33
Friends, 182, 235
Funding, mental health care, 146, 154–158

Gadow, Sally A., 229
Gallagher, Dolores, 49–50, 52
Gastrointestinal problems, 27
Gatz, Margaret, 227

General practitioners, 146, 163
Generalized anxiety disorder, 107, 129
Genetics
    and bipolar disorders, 60
    and depression, 15
    in schizophrenia, 117, 118
Genitourinary dysfunction, 27
George, Linda K., 221
Geriatric psychiatry, 222, 225–226
    fellowship programs, 200–203
Geriatric Psychiatry, 222
Geriatric Research, Education, and Clinical
        Centers (GRECCs), 164, 180, 199–200
Gerontological Society of America (GSA),
        181–182
Gerontology
    clinical, 223
    organizations for, 179–182
Grant, Leslie A., 225
GRECCs. *See* Geriatric Research, Education,
    and Clinical Centers
Greist, John H., 231–232
GSA. *See* Gerontological Society of America
*A Guide to Alzheimer's Disease: For
        Families, Spouses, and Friends*, 235
Gwyther, Lisa P., 224

Haldol, 120
Hallucinations, 73, 89, 105, 110
    and delirium, 87
    in delusional disorders, 113
    in schizophrenia, 112, 117
    as symptom of major depression, 10, 11
    treatment for, 119
Haloperidol, 120
Handbook of Aging and the Social Sciences,
        221
Handbook of Clinical Gerontology, 223
*A Handbook of Geriatric
        Psychopharmacology*, 224
Handbook of Mental Health and Aging, 222
Handbook of the Psychology of Aging, 222
Hansen, Mary, 235
Hardening of the arteries, 69
Haug, Marie R., 222
Health maintenance organizations (HMOs),
        145, 152
Health problems, as cause of depression, 19,
        27–28
Heart problems, 27. *See also* Cardiac disease
Helpful Facts about Depressive Disorders, 242

*The Hidden Victims of Alzheimer's Disease:
        Families under Stress*, 228
High blood pressure, 27
    medication for, 16, 28
History, patient, 27–28, 87
HMOs. *See* Health maintenance
    organizations
Home Care with the Alzheimer Patient,
        236–237
Hooyman, Nancy R., 234, 235
Hospitalization, 153
    as cause of lung disorder, 79
    for schizophrenia, 124
    for substance use problems, 109, 142
    See also Hospitals; Inpatients
Hospitals, 146, 163
    Medicare payments to, 155–156
    psychiatric, 153, 232
    state, 154
    university-affiliated, 164
*How You Can Help: A Guide for Families of
        Psychiatric Hospital Patients*, 232
Huntington's disease, 83
Hydergine, 94
Hypertension, and monoamine oxidase
        inhibitors, 41
Hypnotics, dependence on, 108, 109, 135,
        141, 142
Hypomania, 5, 59
Hypotension, orthostatic, 38–39, 121
Hypothyroidism, 62

Identity, with work role, 30
*If You Have Alzheimer's Disease: What You
        Should Know, What You Can Do*, 237
Illusions, 73, 87
In Care of: Families and Their Elders (video),
        247
Inderal, 132
Infarcts, 75, 82. *See also* Strokes
Infection
    as cause of delirium, 79
    as cause of dementia, 84
Information on Lithium, 242
Inpatients
    bipolar disorder treatment, 64
    care system for, 146, 150, 153–154
    depression treatment, 55–57
Insomnia, as symptom of major depression, 9
Institutions, for mentally ill, 147–148. *See
        also* Hospitals; Nursing homes

Insurance, mental health services, 157
Intoxication, from drugs, 79
Isoxsuprine, 94

Jarvik, Lissy F., 224, 230
Jefferson, James W., 231–232
Jenike, Michael A., 224
Johnson, Colleen L., 225
Judgment, and dementia, 87

Kennedy, John F., 148
Kermis, Marguerite D., 225
Kidneys, lithium's impact on, 62
Kivnik, Helen Q., 229–230
Klerman, Gerald, 65
Knight, Bob, 225
Korpell, Herbert S., 232
Kuru, 81, 83

L-Dopa, 83, 94–95
Language, and dementia, 87
Lazarus, Lawrence W., 225–226
Legal Considerations for Alzheimer's Disease, 237
Let's Talk Facts About: Anxiety Disorders, 237
Let's Talk Facts About: Depression, 237
Let's Talk Facts About: Manic-Depressive Disorder, 238
Let's Talk Facts About: Mental Health of the Elderly, 238
Let's Talk Facts About: Mental Illness: There Are a Lot of Troubled People, 238
Let's Talk Facts About: Obsessive-Compulsive Disorder, 238
Let's Talk Facts About: Phobias, 238
Let's Talk Facts About: Schizophrenia, 238
Let's Talk Facts About: Substance Abuse, 238–239
Lewine, Richard R. J., 231
Lewinsohn, Peter M., 232
Lewis, Myrna I., 223, 233
Life issues, 29
Lithium, 242
    as antidepressant, 42
    for bipolar disorder, 61–65
    and mood disorders, 5, 16
Living skills, daily, 90
Long-term care facilities, 146, 154
Lorazepam, 131

The Loss of Self: A Family Resource for the Care of Alzheimer's Disease and Related Disorders, 233–234
Loxapine succinate, 120
Loxitane, 120
Lung disorder, chronic, 79
Lurie, Elinor E., 226
Lustbader, Wendy, 234

Mace, Nancy L., 234
Magnetic resonance imaging (MRI) scan, 118
Major depression, 3, 119
    characteristics of, 8–11
Managing with Alzheimer's Disease (video), 247–248
Manic depression. *See* Bipolar disorder
Manic episodes, 4, 6
    in bipolar disorder, 57–60
    in delusional disorders, 114
    treatment of, 63
Manpower, 158
MAO inhibitors. *See* Monoamine oxidase inhibitors
Marks, Isaac M., 232
Medicaid, 146, 156–158
Medical centers, university-affiliated, 164
Medical examination, and diagnosis, 89–90
Medical problems, evaluation for, 27–28, 56
Medicare, 146, 151, 154–156
    funding problems, 157–158
Medication, 224, 240, 243, 248
    abuse of, 140, 141
    anti-psychotic, 148
    for anxiety disorder, 131–134
    for bipolar disorder, 5
    as cause of depression, 28–29
    for dysthymia, 4
    for major depression, 3
    monitoring, 142–143
    for mood disorders, 16
    psychotropic, 34
    See also Drugs; Pharmacological treatment
Medication and Dementia (video), 248
Medicines. *See* Drugs; Medication; Pharmacological treatment
Melancholic depression, 11
Mellaril, 120
Memory, loss of, 68–69, 73, 86, 234, 237
Memory and Aging, 237

Mental Disorders of the Aging Research
    Branch, 186
*Mental Health and Aging: Programs and
    Evaluations,* 227
Mental Health Association of Southeastern
    Pennsylvania, 188
Mental health care, 145, 240
*Mental Health Consultations in Nursing
    Homes,* 228
*Mental Health in Late Life: The Adaptive
    Process,* 225
Mental Health Practice with the Elderly,
    223–224
Mental illness, 238, 243
    care of, 147–149
    and family, 231
    pamphlets on, 239
    services for, 226
Mental Illness Is Everybody's Business, 239
Meprobamate, 133
Metabolic disturbance
    as cause of delirium, 79
    as cause of dementia, 84
Metastases, 84
Methylphenidate, 94
MID. *See* Multi-infarct dementia
Miller, Nancy E., 226
Milt, Harry, 232–233
Miltown, 133
Ministers, 163
Mixed dementia, 78
Moban, 120
Molindone HC1, 120
Monoamine oxidase (MAO) inhibitors, to
    treat depression, 40–41, 95
Mood disorders, 239
    and psychotic symptoms, 119
    and schizophrenia, 112
*Mood Disorders: Depression and Manic
    Depression,* 239
MRI. *See* Magnetic resonance imaging scan
Multi-infarct dementia (MID), 68, 75, 82, 101
    characteristics of, 76–77, 87
    frequency of, 78
    treatment of, 93
Multiple personality disorder, 111
Munoz, Ricardo F., 232
Mutual help, 243. *See also* Self-help

NAAA. *See* National Association of Area
    Agencies on Aging

NAMI. *See* National Alliance for the
    Mentally Ill
NASUA. *See* National Association of State
    Units on Aging
NASW. *See* National Association of Social
    Workers
National Academy of Certified Clinical
    Mental Health Counselors, 167
National Alliance for the Mentally Ill
    (NAMI), 182, 239
National Association of Area Agencies on
    Aging (NAAA), 183
National Association of Social Workers
    (NASW), 183–184
    chapter offices, 205–208
National Association of State Units on Aging
    (NASUA), state organizations, 208–213
National Council of Community Mental
    Health Centers (NCCMHC), 184–185,
    226
    model programs, 203–205
National Depressive and Manic Depressive
    Association (NDMDA), 185
National Institute of Mental Health
    (NIMH), 186
    pamphlets, 241–244
National Institute on Aging (NIA)
    Information Center, 186–187
    pamphlets, 239–241
    research funding, 188
National Mental Health Association, 187,
    244
    affiliated divisions and chapters, 213–215
National Mental Health Consumers
    Self-Help Clearinghouse, 188
Navane, 120
NCCMHC. *See* National Council of
    Community Mental Health Centers
NDMDA. *See* National Depressive and
    Manic Depressive Association
Neuroleptics, 63, 161
    for dementia, 95–96
    for schizophrenia, 106, 119–124
Neuropsychology, testing, 88
Neurosyphilis, 83
NIA. *See* National Institute on Aging
NIMH. *See* National Institute of Mental
    Health
Normal pressure hydrocephalus (NPH), 84
NPH. *See* Normal pressure hydrocephalus
Nurses, psychiatric, 166

The Nursing Home in American Society, 225
Nursing homes, 145, 150, 154, 225, 228,
    235
    Alzheimer's patients in, 224
    Medicaid, 156–157
    problems in, 161–162
Nutrition
    alcoholism and, 141
    and dementia, 84

Obsessions, 107, 128
Obsessive-compulsive disorder, 107, 128,
    134, 238
O'Conner, Kathleen, 227
Older Americans Act, 153
Organic brain syndrome, 69
Organic mental disorders, 67–68, 72
    types of, 75–77
Organic mental syndromes, 67, 72
    types of, 73–75
Organizations
    national, 175–188
    state and local, 188–219
Orr, Nancy K., 228
Orthostatic change
    with antidepressants, 38–39
    with neuroleptics, 121
Outpatients
    bipolar disorder treatment, 64
    care system for, 145, 150–153
    depression treatment, 54–57

Pain, 29, 79
Pamphlets, 235
    Alzheimer's Association, 236–237
    American Psychiatric Association,
        237–239
    National Alliance for the Mentally Ill, 239
    National Institute of Mental Health,
        241–244
    National Institute on Aging, 239–241
    National Mental Health Association, 244
Panic disorder, 106–107, 130, 243
    characteristics, 125–126
    treatment for, 133
Papaverine, 94
Papolos, Demitri, 239
Paranoia, 116
Paraphrenia, 116–118
*Parentcare: A Commonsense Guide for
    Adult Children,* 230

Parents, 229, 230
Paresis, 83
Parkinson's disease, 27, 75, 83, 95
Pentylenetetrazol, 94
Perphenazine, 120
Personality, changes in, 75, 83, 87
Personality disorders, 118
PET. *See* Positron emission tomography
    scan
Pharmacological treatment
    for delirium and reversible dementia,
        92–93
    for depression, 34, 57
    geriatric, 224, 227
    for irreversible dementia, 93–96
    See also Drugs; Medication
Phobias, 134, 232–233, 238, 243. *See also*
    Anxiety disorders; specific types
Physical examinations, 27–28
Physical illness, 30
Physician, family, 163
Physostigmine, 94
Pick's disease, 75, 78, 83
Pipradrol, 94
Plain Talk about Aging, 242
Plain Talk about Mutual Help Groups, 243
Poorhouses, 147, 148
Positron emission tomography (PET) scan,
    118
Post, Felix, 32
Powell, Lenore S., 234
Presenile dementia, 77
Priests, 163
Primary degenerative dementia. *See*
    Alzheimer's disease
Private practitioners
    Medicare, 155
    mental health care, 145, 151
Problems, family skills for solving, 100–101
*Progress Report on Alzheimer's Disease,
    Volume II,* 241
Project SHARE, 188
Prolixin, 120
Propranolol, 132
Prothero, Joyce, 227
Prozac, 42
Pseudodementia, 32–33, 84, 85, 87, 93
Psoriasis, and lithium treatment, 62
Psychiatric institutions, 145, 232
Psychiatrists, 151, 166
    organizations for, 176, 178

Psychiatry, geriatric, 200–203, 222, 225–226
Psychoactive substance abuse, 137
Psychoactive substance dependence, 108, 136–137
Psychodynamics, and depression, 20–21
Psychologists, 161, 166
Psychology, 222, 228
Psychomotor agitation, as symptom of major depression, 9
Psychomotor retardation, as symptom of major depression, 9
Psychotherapists, 167
Psychotherapy, 225
    behavioral and cognitive, 49–52
    for bipolar disorder, 5, 64
    for clinical depression, 44–46, 57
    couple, 52–53
    for dysthymia, 4
    family, 53–54
    group, 52
    for major depression, 3
    nursing homes, 161
    psychodynamic, 48–49
    reminiscence, 49
    supportive, 46–48
Psychotherapy with Older Adults, 225
Psychotic, 10
Psychotic symptoms, 105, 110
    evaluation of, 119
    paranoia in, 116–117
    in schizophrenia, 111
Psychotropic medication
    for depression, 34, 36–42
    function of, 35–36

Q & A: Alzheimer's Disease, 241

Rabbis, 163
Rabins, Peter V., 234
Rapport, establishing, 24–25
Reisberg, Barry, 102, 235
Religious organizations, mental health services, 153, 163
Reminiscence therapy, 49
Reserpine, and depression, 16, 28
Residential care facilities, 150
Respite care, 164
Retirement, 20
Richards, Mary, 235

Rosow, Irving, 19
Roth, Martin, 32, 116–117

Salzman, Carl, 227
Schaie, K. Warner, 222, 230
Schizoaffective disorder, and schizophrenia, 112
Schizophrenia, 89, 226, 238, 239, 243, 244
    causes of, 117–118
    characteristics of, 105–106
    definition of, 111–113
    evaluation of, 119
    frequency of, 117
    in later life, 116–117
    treatment of, 119–124
Schizophrenia, 244
Schizophrenia: Questions and Answers, 243
Schizophrenia and Aging: Schizophrenia, Paranoia, and Schizophreniform Disorders in Later Life, 226
Second-generation antidepressants, 41–42
Secondary amines, 37, 39
Sedation
    with antidepressants, 39
    with benzodiazepines, 131
    with neuroleptics, 121
Sedatives, dependence on, 108, 109, 135, 141, 142
Self
    loss of, 233–234
    sense of, 68–69
Self-help, 164–165, 243
    clearinghouses for, 215–218
    organizations for, 188, 218–219
Senile dementia, 69, 77
Senility, 69, 240
Services, 226
    community mental health centers, 148–149, 226–227
    coordination of, 159–160
    for dementia patients, 98–99
    finding, 162–165
    mental health, 223–224, 241–242
    outpatient, 55, 150–153
    reluctance to use, 160–161
    supportive, 153, 177
    use of, 165–169
    See also Organizations
Serving the Elderly: A Mental Health Resource Guide, 226–227

Serving the Mentally Ill Elderly: Problems and Perspectives, 226
Shock therapy. *See* Electroconvulsive therapy
Side effects
    of antidepressants, 38–40
    of benzodiazepines, 131–132
    of lithium treatment, 62
    of neuroleptics, 63, 95, 121–122
Simple phobia, 107, 127, 130
Skills, self-care, 148
Skinner, B. F., 230–231
Sleep
    medication for, 29
    as symptom of major depression, 9
Sloane, R. Bruce, 222
Small, Gary, 230
Smith-DiJulio, Kathy, 235
Smyer, Michael A., 227–228
Social phobias, 107, 127
Social roles, 19–20
Social service organizations, 145
Social skills
    and depression, 22–23, 232
    and psychotic illness, 118
Social workers, 166
    organizations for, 184, 205–208
Society
    aging and, 221
    response to mental disorders, 147–148
Speech, schizophrenia and, 112
Stelazine, 120
Stigma: A Lack of Awareness and Understanding, 244
Stress, 244
    and anxiety, 130
    and depression, 14, 17–20
    family, 228
Stress: A Fact of Life, 244
Strokes, 27, 75, 83. *See also* Multi-infarct dementia
Substance use disorders, 108–109, 238–239
    causes of, 138–140
    definition of, 135–137
    evaluation of, 140–142
    frequency of, 137–138
    treatment of, 142–143
Suicide, 243
    factors in, 30–32
    and major depression, 3, 10
Support groups, 248–249
    for caregivers, 101, 164

Swan, James H., 226
Syndrome, defined, 67, 72

Tacrine, 94
Taking Care: Supporting Older People and Their Families, 234
Talking with Your Aging Parents, 229
Tardive dyskinesia (TD), and neuroleptics, 63, 95, 122–123
TD. *See* Tardive dyskinesia
Tegretol, 63
Tertiary amines, 37, 39
Tetrahydroaminoacridine (THA), 94
THA. *See* Tetrahydroaminoacridine
Therapy
    behavioral, 133–134
    contextual, 232–233
    occupational, 147–148
There Were Times, Dear (video/film), 248–249
Thinking patterns
    and delirium, 87
    and dementia, 86
    and depression, 23–24
    negative, 50–52
Thioridazine, 120
Thiothixene, 120
The 36-Hour Day: A Family Guide to Caring for Persons with Alzheimer's Disease, Related Illnesses, and Memory Loss in Later Life, 98
Thompson, Larry, 49–50, 52
Thorazine, 120
Thought disorder, 105, 110, 119
Thyroid disease, 27
To Be Old and Sad: Understanding Depression in the Elderly, 233
Tomlinson, B. E., 71
Toxicity, drug and alcohol, 142–143
Training, 158
    on aging, 186
    nursing homes, 161
Tranquilizers, 95, 240
    major, 63
    See also specific names
Trazodone, 42
Treatment
    for Alzheimer's disease, 186–187, 224
    for anxiety disorders, 107–108, 131–134, 232–233
    for bipolar disorder, 61–65

Treatment *(continued)*
  costs of, 167
  for delirium and dementia, 92–101
  for delusional disorders, 119, 123
  for depression, 34–54, 231, 242
  effectiveness, 56–57
  manic episodes, 63
  outcome of, 168
  procedures of, 168
  review of, 169
  of schizophrenia, 119–124
  settings, 54–56
  substance use disorders, 109, 142–143
Treatment for the Alzheimer Patient: The Long Haul, 224
Trifluoperazine HC1, 120
Trilafon, 120
Tumors
  as cause of delirium, 79
  as cause of dementia, 84

Understanding and Coping with Dementia (video), 249
Useful Information On . . . Alzheimer's Disease, 243
Useful Information On . . . Medications for Mental Illness, 243
Useful Information On . . . Phobias and Panic, 243
Useful Information On . . . Suicide, 243

VA. *See* Department of Veterans Affairs
Valium, 131
Vasodilators, 94
Vasopressin (Vp), 94
Vaughan, M. E., 230–231
Videocassettes, 244–250
Viruses, 27, 81
Vital Involvement in Old Age, 229–230
Vp. *See* Vasopressin

Weissmann, Myrna, 65
Wellbutrin, 42
We're Not Alone (video), 249–250
Wernicke-Korsakoff's syndrome, 141
What Does It Mean To Grow Old? Reflections from the Humanities, 229
What Is Schizophrenia?, 239
Why Survive? Being Old in America, 228–229
Willis, Sherry L., 230
Wilson's disease, 83
Winograd, Carol H., 224
Withdrawal symptoms, 137, 142
Work role, 20, 30

Youngren, Mary Ann, 232
Your Phobia: Understanding Your Fears through Contextual Therapy, 232–233

Zane, Manuel D., 232–233
Zarit, Judy M., 228
Zarit, Steven, 99–100, 228
Zeiss, Antonette M., 232